THE FEASIBILITY OF FERTILITY PLANNING

THE FEASIBILITY OF FERTILITY PLANNING

Micro Perspectives

EDITED BY

T. SCARLETT EPSTEIN

AND

DARRELL JACKSON

Institute of Development Studies,
University of Sussex

PERGAMON PRESS

OXFORD · NEW YORK · TORONTO · SYDNEY · PARIS · FRANKFURT

U.K.	Pergamon Press Ltd., Headington Hill Hall, Oxford OX3 0BW, England
U.S.A.	Pergamon Press Inc., Maxwell House, Fairview Park, Elmsford, New York 10523, U.S.A.
CANADA	Pergamon of Canada Ltd., 75 The East Mall, Toronto, Ontario, Canada
AUSTRALIA	Pergamon Press (Aust.) Pty. Ltd., 19a Boundary Street, Rushcutters Bay, N.S.W. 2011, Australia
FRANCE	Pergamon Press SARL, 24 Rue des Ecoles, 75240 Paris, Cedex 05, France
WEST GERMANY	Pergamon Press GmbH, 6242 Kronberg-Taunus, Pferdstrasse 1, Frankfurt-am-Main, West Germany

First edition 1977

Library of Congress Catalog Card Number 77-76600

In order to make this volume available as economically and rapidly as possible the authors' typescripts have been reproduced in their original form. This method unfortunately has its typographical limitations but it is hoped that they in no way distract the reader.

Printed in Great Britain by A. Wheaton & Co., Exeter

ISBN 0 08 021452 5 (Hard cover)
ISBN 0 08 021837 7 (Flexi cover)

CONTENTS

LIST OF PLATES

ACKNOWLEDGEMENTS

The research project from which this book originates is financed by the World Bank, the Population Council, and the Ministry of Overseas Development, England, to whom major acknowledgements are due.* We are grateful for the continued encouragement which these institutions have given us, and particularly for their willingness to support - in this era of scarce research resources - the type of cross-cultural study which we believe has much to contribute towards a genuine understanding of crucial Third World issues.

Acknowledgements must also be made to the Institute of Development Studies, University of Sussex, which has sponsored the project since its first tentative hypothesis three years ago, and which continues to provide a stimulating multi-disciplinary forum for the debate of many of the issues raised in this volume. Amongst our many colleagues and friends there, thanks must go to Robert Cassen and Mick Moore in particular for allowing us to draw so generously on their considerable experience in the field of population studies.

We would similarly like to express our gratitude to those colleagues in the four fieldwork countries who have acted as informal consultants, and provided a host of useful insights into the particularities of the eight research locations. Dr. T.N. Madan (Institute of Economic Growth, Delhi), C. Narayanasamy (Agricultural Research and Training Institute, Colombo), Dr. Ranjit Senaratne (Marga Institute, Colombo), Dr. Philip Mbithi and J.H. van Doorne (University of Nairobi), and Dr. E.J. Nwosu (University of Nigeria), have all given much time and energy in collaborating with our team. Without their help the work of the project and the analyses presented here would have been much diminished.

The interim project reports on which this volume is based were originally given as papers at a conference held at the Institute of Development Studies in December 1975. Whilst lack of time has precluded the incorporation of the many genuinely constructive comments made, we would nonetheless like to acknowledge those individuals whose contributions provoked a critical reassessment of certain aspects of the project's methodological and conceptual framework. In particular, Susan Almy, Rudolf Andorka, Jan Breman, Joan Chapman, Timothy King, Geoffrey McNicholl, David Parkin, John Simons and Abe Weisblat managed not only to survive the rigours which such conferences inevitably entail, but also to consistently point us in fresh and rewarding directions, which we hope will be reflected in the quality of the final research reports. Additionally, Jayantha Perera provided a useful record of the conference proceedings.

* The views expressed in this book are not necessarily endorsed by these institutions.

Gratitude must also be expressed to Tarzie Vittachi of the United Nations Fund for Population Activities for being generally supportive of our endeavours, and also for permission to reprint the chapters by Monica Das Gupta and Joseph Ssennyonga, which originally appeared in the UNFPA journal *Populi*, Volume 3, Numbers 1 and 2 respectively. We are similarly grateful for Robert Maxwell's expression of interest in publishing this volume.

Peter Kane provided valuable editorial assistance, and Rosemary Watts, whose typing abilities reflect only a fraction of her many accomplishments, must take much of the credit for the production of this book. Her cheerful commitment to the means and ends of the project is rapidly becoming a phenomenon deserving of study in its own right.

Finally, we would like to record our indebtedness to the people in the eight villages who were the unwitting victims of our insatiable thirst for knowledge. Many friendships were made which transcended - and fortunately, perhaps, at times supplanted - the role of the social scientist as an objective and impassive observer. In terms of wisdom exchanged there can be little doubt that we were the principal beneficiaries.

Whilst we have no illusions that our research will in any way enhance the quality of their lives, we would like to dedicate this book to them as a measure of our gratitude for their kindness, and in the hope that the knowledge gleaned from studying their role within a system whose origins and forces are often obscure, will ultimately contribute to changes which will enable them to shape that system themselves in accordance with their own needs and aims.

T. SCARLETT EPSTEIN
DARRELL JACKSON
Sussex, November 1976

PART 1

INTRODUCTION

CHAPTER 1

PARADIGMS AND PERSPECTIVES — A CROSS-CULTURAL APPROACH TO POPULATION GROWTH AND RURAL POVERTY

INTRODUCTION

The censuses of 1960 confirmed the long-held belief of demographic observers that population growth in most, if not all, Third World countries was increasing at a hitherto unprecedented rate. This realisation was rapidly followed by Malthusian forebodings about the threat of absolute world over-population, whilst at the same time serious concern was expressed over the seeming imminence and inevitability of other global threats to the rich countries' future living standards, notably resource depletion and environmental deterioration.

The alarms were officially sounded in the 1960 resolutions of the First U.N. Development Decade, and thereafter the 'population problem' took its place among the other major variables - employment, education, income distribution, agrarian reform, etc. - which were identified as key issues determining the structure of poverty and inequality within Third World countries.

Much of the research being carried out at the time (e.g. Enke, 1967) seemed to justify this belief. When presented with the proposition that 'The addition to income per head in a poor country caused by spending £100 on birth prevention is, at very least, fifteen times the addition to income per head from the best alternative use of £100' (Lipton, 1971:48), large scale investment by donor agencies in these new techniques appeared to be a rational - if not imperative - strategy.

The initial response of most developed country governments and aid organisations to the population problem was to launch massive schemes involving the export of new birth-control technology, in the hope that indigenous governments would distribute these techniques within the framework of a more or less integrated national family planning programme. The irony that the problem had been directly created by the application of Western medical technology (particularly through the almost total eradication of malaria), which upset the fertility/mortality balance by significantly reducing mortality rates, was coupled with the belief that the solution was to be similarly found in technology, i.e. the new birth-control techniques developed in the early 1960's - notably the pill, loop and IUD. It was hoped that these modern means of contraception would restore the balance by reducing fertility levels and slowing down the prevailing population growth rates of 2-3% per annum.

This response, which was part of the general tendency to treat high population growth rates as a problem in an absolute sense, and as a significant potential threat which might thwart development strategies, was consistent with the general tenor of most development thinking during that period. Dominated by macro-economic perspectives, the writings of the time abound with grim prophecies about the inhibiting effects of the population explosion on the economic growth potential of 'underdeveloped' economies. Whether it was a question of the 'take-off' point not being reached (Rostow, 1960), or the threat of economic development efforts being entirely frustrated (Myrdal, 1970), the problems which rapid population growth posed tended to be reduced to simplistic statements based on aggregate statistics: if the population was increasing at a greater rate than the national income, then it could not be said that development was taking place. This approach - of using national income data as indicators of development - was supported by the notions which led to the target of 5% growth rates in GNP set during the first development decade.

Although the confusion which followed from the definition of 'development' as economic growth was relatively short-lived, the post-war stress on growth maximisation policies, which it is now claimed implicitly assumed a 'trickle-down' effect to rural areas, obscured the identification of genuine development indicators in the very place where development was *not* taking place and where at least 70% of the Third World's population live - the rural areas. Seers (1969) suggested that development should be considered in relation to the variable levels of three main factors: poverty (basic nutritional and associated needs), employment, and equality - the latter being pursued as an end in itself. He then pointed out the inherent fallacy in using aggregate data such as national income statistics as development indicators, namely that it is quite possible for per capita income to be increasing in a period of national economic expansion, whilst at the same time poverty also increases and the gap between rich and poor grows larger. On a national or sub-national level we must therefore assume that the measurement of development implies looking at distributional as well as growth factors.

This approach to development generally has had important consequences at both policy and research levels.

Taking policy first, it is now generally accepted that the measures taken to implement the recommendations expressed during the first development decade had virtually no impact on retarding fertility rates. The insistence of rich-country governments and other agencies on family planning as the sole panacea was not only misplaced as a realistic policy instrument, it also succeeded in creating suspicions in the minds of Third World planners that such a strategy was little more than a thinly-veiled attempt to protect the interests of the policy instigators who had suddenly awoken to the threats - economic and political - which rapid population growth seemed to present.

On a policy level it was not merely a question of 'too little too late', but rather a genuine misunderstanding of the causes of high fertility and consequently of the measures necessary to effect changes. It could well be argued that, given the effect on mortality rates of the new medical technology, one could not expect immediate results from a family planning campaign due to the adaptive lag which precedes the realisation that declining infant mortality makes it less necessary to have large numbers of children in order to ensure the survival of a few. Similarly, it has been argued that whilst the techniques of family limitation were quite adequate, effective implementation of the programmes was restricted by a shortage of trained medical staff. Again it has been suggested that the physiological effects of some techniques destroyed people's confidence in their efficacy. However, all these reasons given for the relative failure of family planning programmes rest on two assumptions that have been shown to be palpably false, namely, that techniques of fertility control were previously unknown in traditional societies, and secondly that those concerned actually *wanted* to reduce their fertility. Since the means already existed, the realisation had to be faced that people still wanted large families, and it was equally evident that many of the existing research methodologies and theories were incapable of providing explanations of this fundamental point.

It should perhaps be stressed here that it is not intended to relegate the role of family planning to a subordinate or peripheral status. Clearly the technological improvements of the last two decades have been of immense importance in providing safe and assured methods of family size limitation. Rather it is the stress on the pre-eminence of family planning which is being questioned and a plea for the recognition that the use of such techniques constitutes a necessary but not sufficient condition for effecting changes in demographic trends. Since the early 70s many Third World governments have included population reduction targets based on the use of new family limitation techniques in their development plans, which is obviously an important step forward. Fortunately our state of knowledge has progressed to the extent that it is now recognised that 'Within the population field, there is a broad concensus that both development programs and family planning programs are necessary, but that neither alone is sufficient to bring about long-term societal regulation of fertility trends' (Arnold et al, 1975:11).

If the development of effective and realistic policy measures has a general tendency to lag behind changes in the real world, it has been accompanied by the absence of research frameworks which can adequately define, measure and provide causal explanations of the problem in hand.[1] This seems to be particularly the case with population studies, and in some respects these inadequacies derive from the phenomena being studied. Whilst it may be feasible to develop theories and design models on the

---

1. There are of course other constraints. Roy cites the work of Plato, Malthus, Stuart Mill and Marx in stressing that 'population policies historically have been tied to social and political ideologies and have shifted from one base to another' (1975:96)

assumption that economic man will generally act rationally in his assumed pursuit of maximisation, it is somewhat less feasible to make similarly rational inferences about the motivations and behaviour of people involved in the various aspects of child-bearing and child-rearing. In the latter case *'ceteris'* are not always *'paribus'* and the variables are less susceptible to purely quantitative analysis.

Even so, one of the legacies inherited from the post-war growth maximisation/aggregate measurement approach has been the perpetuation of attempts to apply the tools of macro and micro-economic analysis within an area where their predictive and explanatory power appears to be limited. As Greenwood (1976) has demonstrated, there are still vast tracts of land within the social scientist's territory which obstinately defy explanations based on formalist assumptions about man's behaviour, and predictions derived from statistically aggregated - but nonetheless mythical - average man.

At the macro level, the types of statistics and analyses suggested by the need for the long term national plans formulated in the 60's were inevitably based on such readily quantifiable variables as capital/output ratios, man/land ratios and fertility and mortality rates. These data in turn are amenable to cross-section analyses, projections and other sophisticated statistical techniques. Whilst few would deny the importance of these methods, it became rapidly evident when serious attention was first paid to the determinants of continued high fertility, that they were not sufficiently comprehensive to throw light on the complexity of the phenomena observed. It was felt by many at the time that the prospect of demographic transitions in the Third World - whereby the characteristic changes associated with industrialisation involve higher child-rearing costs, and hence significant reduction in fertility rates - obviated the need for closer scrutiny of the mechanisms affecting family size at the micro level.

When the shift to micro level research did occur, much of the theory and methods of the earlier approach were simply transferred to this new level. The now extensive field of studies based on micro-economic theories of fertility determination is too large to be covered here in detail, but the work of Becker (1960), Easterlin (1969), Espenshade (1972) and Namboodiri (1972) may be mentioned as examples of attempts to explain fertility behaviour on the basis of the perceived costs and benefits of child bearing and rearing.

Now the assumption that a reasonably high degree of rationality is involved in the family size decision-making process is quite evidently a reasonable one for societies in which people can perceive the options open to them and are in a position to choose between them, and it is this assumption which underpins the postulations of demographic transition theory. Similarly, one must attribute an equal degree of rationality to those making family size decisions in the Third World, since there is no reason to believe that they are any less aware of the costs and benefits than their urban or rich country counterparts. One is thus forced to conclude that the landless and undernourished millions who make up such a significant percentage of the Third World's population actually *want* large numbers of children. Given that pre- and post-natal methods of fertility control have long been practised in most traditional societies, it should not perhaps have taken us so long to reach this conclusion. One must therefore question the means by which this conclusion was ultimately reached.

Without entering into the formalist-substantivist debate, the relatively small number of micro-level studies conducted to date suggest that the tools of formal economic analysis are more applicable to market-integrated societies, and that consequently different or modified methods must be used to analyse behaviour in non-market integrated societies, which would encompass much of the Third World. This is apparent since many of the 'benefits' derived from large numbers of children are not direct economic benefits; socio-political considerations relating to status and prestige are also influential factors, quite apart from the inherent psychological and emotional satisfactions. Equally, it would appear that the motivation for having a large family is often not the maximisation of gains, but rather a consequence of the normative pressures arising from the institutional and cultural environment.

There is not necessarily a contradiction between the formalist and the substantivist approach, and the fact that a consensus is emerging from different disciplines on the notion of the value of children is an encouraging example of the complementarity of seemingly opposed perspectives. Recently the inadequacies of a purely economistic analysis have been partially remedied by the growing interest shown by sociologists, anthropologists, psychologists and demographers in the micro-level determinants of family size and structure.[2]

This multi-disciplinary approach is central to the research project on which this book is based, but before turning to an elaboration of the project it would be useful to consider briefly recent changes in development thinking generally, and more particularly in the field of population policy, which have greatly influenced the construction and implementation of the project.

A New Realism

Taking general changes in development thinking first, it may well be that the mid-1970's will be seen as the watershed which marked significant departures from previous orthodoxies.[3] These

2. This complementarity has been examined in greater depth by Dyson (1975).
3. For an elaboration of this discussion see e.g. Ranis (1976) and Jolly (1976).

changes followed the realisation that the encouraging economic performance of most Third World countries in the previous two decades had obscured an increasing divergence both between and within these countries. It became necessary to reconsider the wisdom of many of the old orthodoxies, such as growth maximisation, high investment in heavy industry and the allocation of resources where the rate of return is highest. Effective policies had to take account of the growing distinction between Third World countries which were either rich in natural resources or were characterised by high labour intensive output/export structures (e.g. Taiwan and Korea) on the one hand, and areas such as India, Bangladesh, some Central African and Latin American countries which had neither of these 'benefits' and whose problems were further exacerbated by the recent increases in oil, fertiliser and food prices.

Much of the new orthodoxy which has arisen in response to these and other changes is contained in the report of the International Labour Office submitted to the Tripartite World Conference on Employment, Income Distribution and Social Progress and the International Division of Labour (ILO, 1976). Briefly, a set of *basic needs* has been identified, whose two main elements are certain minimum requirements such as adequate food, shelter and clothing, and secondly the provision of such essential services as sanitation, public transport, health and educational facilities. It is of particular relevance to the present study that 'a basic-needs oriented policy implies the participation of the people in making the decisions which affect them' (*op. cit.*: 32). This point will be taken up at length in the ensuing discussion of the project's interim findings.

The provision of such needs involves the identification of target groups, who would benefit from a series of shifts in investment from physical to human capital, from urban to rural development, from capital intensive to labour intensive activities, and from the production of non-essential consumer goods to essential ones. Such a strategy stresses the need to maintain economic growth rates, whilst at the same time ensuring that asset transfer from the rich to the poor is increased significantly.

The relevance of the new orthodoxy to population studies is twofold. First, the swing away from the neo-Malthusian approach is emphasised by the assumption that the provision of such basic requirements will reduce the need for large families and provide an incentive for fertility declines: '..... development strategies aimed at reducing social inequalities and at the rapid and widespread satisfaction of basic needs and the consequent raising of aspirations may be very effective in changing family attitudes to family size (*op. cit.*: 60). Second, much of this thinking accords with recent changes in the field of population studies, as evidenced by the positions taken by many countries at the World Population Conference held in Bucharest in 1974.

Before examining these changes in more detail, it is worth noting that although the Basic Needs report implicitly assumes the importance of population growth, no policy recommendations are forthcoming. The brief section devoted to the matter concludes - somewhat tamely in the context of such a bold attack on injustice and inequality - that 'much further research is needed' (*op. cit.*: 60). Additionally, whilst one is loath to criticise such brave rhetoric, it must be remembered that implementation of the strategies outlined is constrained by the shifting sands of political reality. It is difficult to envisage such changes occurring in the near future, given the present nature of this reality in many of the countries where these changes are most urgently required.

Turning now to the parallel shifts in thought which finally surfaced at the Bucharest Conference, one fundamental point on which a reasonable degree of consensus emerged was the rejection of a previously long held assumption that population growth was a problem *per se*, and that consequently studies of the 'problem' should treat population growth as an independent variable. This assumption stemmed largely from the notion that capital/output and capital/labour ratios were fixed, and that, since significant capital or technological changes could not be hoped for, it was necessary to concentrate on the possibility of a rapid decline in population growth, the latter being seen as the only variable amenable to change. At the same time rapid population growth rates were seen as a factor constraining potential national income growth and full employment. Rather than exploring ways of maximising the efficiency of an increasing labour force, macro analyses tended to focus on the damaging consequences of high fertility rates. According to this familiar argument, high fertility leads to an increased dependency ratio, which in turn creates more sharing of available resources and hence less saving and capital accumulation. Further, a higher proportion of these reduced savings is required for the provision of social services, thus diverting capital towards non-productive investment. It was this perspective in particular which was felt to be an unacceptable starting point for discussion of population matters.

Yet perhaps the real value of the Bucharest Conference lies in the fact that for the first time population-related issues were brought firmly into the political arena. Whilst professionals in the area of population studies expressed dismay at the subsequent exclusion of their own academic expertise, they cannot now seriously afford to ignore the national and international exigencies of political reality. The spectrum of ideological dissension at Bucharest was wide, and one of the polar positions was particularly disheartening for students of population problems - namely that such problems did not exist; insofar as they were perceived to exist by some observers, they could only be ameliorated by internationally co-ordinated attempts at raising the social and economic living standards of Third World populations, such as the much-heralded New International Economic Order.

The present study welcomes such disruptions of the notion of 'population problems', the more so because many of the similar sentiments expressed are fundamentally embodied in the assumptions and interim conclusions of this research project. In view of the importance of the Bucharest conference in influencing on-going and future population research, and by way of introduction to our project itself, it will be pertinent to outline briefly some of the principal issues which emerged, and subsequently relate them to our project's theoretical and methodological perspectives. Apart from the points raised above, there are nine other main areas of congruence between the more or less consensually agreed recommendations of the conference,[4] and our project's orientation. The first point - which was made by default and hence was implicit - was that discussion of population issues should not focus solely on technical aspects such as family planning programmes, distribution of contraceptives, purely demographic research, etc., but should attempt to place these factors within the framework of national development strategies. Second, that the need for social and economic development and a more equitable distribution of wealth should be stressed. Similarly, that analyses of such issues should consider the inter-relationship between population growth and other socio-economic variables. Fourthly, that family planning is not seen as a potential means of speeding up the development process. This relates to the point made earlier that such programmes may be a necessary but not a sufficient condition for bringing about fertility declines and increasing national economic growth rates. Fifth, that the role and status of women is now recognised as a crucial variable influencing fertility decisions, quite apart from the intrinsic human rights aspect. Sixth, that demographic variables are derivative effects of the socio-economic environment to a much greater extent than has hitherto been recognised. The seventh point is embodied in a resolution of the First Committee of the conference, namely that increased agricultural production and the intensification of agrarian reforms should be cardinal points in any development strategy which includes an integrated population policy. Eighth, that the family is perceived as the basic unit both of analysis and of national level decisions. This perspective is fundamental to our project's methodological assumptions since it reflects the belief that the factors affecting fertility decisions are principally understood by micro-level analyses of households and the socio-economic structure within which they operate. Finally, the role of education as a mediating variable both in the family-size decision making process and in the context of national development. Surprisingly this last point did not receive the critical attention which many would argue it deserves. It will be seen that most of the above perspectives are constantly echoed in the chapters which follow.

---

4. It has been argued that the agreed recommendations were often reached after lengthy political manoeuvering and that they were in any event more in the nature of low 'common denominators' rather than receiving wholehearted and widespread support. For an elaboration of this view and a fuller report on the conference see Maudlin et al., 1974.

A Cross-Cultural Study of Population Growth and Rural Poverty

Whilst recent developments such as Bucharest, World Population Year, and the raising of population issues in many policy statements (e.g. the Arusha Declaration) have ensured a need for the continued consideration of population policies - albeit within the framework of an integrated overall strategy - a demand still exists for research which not only explains fertility decisions as one aspect of human behaviour, but also throws up policy recommendations in the form of predictions as to how this behaviour is likely to vary in different social, economic and political structures. A comprehensive approach must therefore include structural as well as more reductionist perspectives. An extreme example of the latter is to be found in the work of Arnold et al. (1975) previously cited. This study attempts to answer the basic question of why people have children, using cross-cultural data derived from a series of interviews and questionnaires. This approach is to be welcomed and is seen as complementary to the work of our own project. The latter seeks answers to the same question, again in a cross-cultural setting, but employing social anthropological techniques of inquiry which involve in-depth case studies.

At the same time a structuralist approach is employed in order to place fertility decisions in a more holistic perspective. Following Kuznets 'the population growth variable is (seen as) significant largely in that it reflects the institutional and social conditions of a country' (1975:19). In this context the present study seeks to analyse the socio-economic variables affecting fertility decisions in different rural strata, the effects of population growth on rural labour supply and income distribution and finally the adaptive capacities of social institutions in the face of population increases. It should be stressed that the following chapters represent the interim results of a four-year project which will be completed towards the end of 1977. The rationale for publishing these inevitably tentative results before all the data have been rigorously analysed lies in the belief that they should be made available to others involved in similar research as soon as possible. This provides an opportunity for critical feedback which can subsequently be incorporated in the final report, as well as being a contribution to the current debate.[5]

Research plan

The present project began in September 1973 when eight doctoral students were selected by the Project Director, Professor Scarlett Epstein, to undertake the research. These researchers,

---

5. A collection of pre-fieldwork theoretical papers by project members has been published as *The Paradox of Poverty: Socio-Economic Aspects of Population Growth*, ed. Epstein and Jackson, Macmillans, Delhi, 1975. Further publications on the project's findings will be available in the near future.

whose work is presented here, are all indigenous to the four countries where fieldwork was carried out - India, Kenya, Nigeria and Sri Lanka. During the initial one year training period at the Institute of Development Studies, Sussex, micro-societies were selected with the help of experts from the relevant countries. A basic criterion in the selection of these societies was that an earlier study had been undertaken at least 25 years previously, in order to provide a data base with a gap of one generation.[6] Further details are provided in Table 1.1.

Table 1.1

Population project fieldwork locations

Researcher	Location	Country
Mukul Dube	Mulkipur	India
Monica Das Gupta	Rampur	India
Vinod Jairath	Ramdaua	India
George Mkangi	Taita-Taveta	Kenya
Joseph Ssennyonga	Viyalo	Kenya
Sammy Onwuazor	Umueke	Nigeria
Newton Gunasinghe	Delumgoda	Sri Lanka
W.M. Tilakaratne	Aluthgama-Bogamuwa	Sri Lanka

The researchers were intentionally drawn from a variety of disciplines, and after a period of training in demographic techniques by Tim Dyson, the project's demographic consultant, and in social anthropological methods, a period of twelve months fieldwork was undertaken. During this and the final period of fieldwork close contact was maintained with Third World institutions, whose personnel acted as informal supervisors of the research. Subsequently the researchers returned to Sussex to prepare papers for a conference held in December 1975. These papers form the basis of the present volume. At the beginning of 1976 a further eight months fieldwork was carried out, after which the team returned to Sussex once more to analyse their data and complete the final project reports.

Methodology

Apart from training in statistical techniques, data analysis methods and more general demographic training, the project methodology draws heavily on the use of survey techniques within a framework of participant observation. A major concern was to evolve a methodology which would provide reliable quantitative

---

6. In this respect we are indebted to Oscar Lewis, K.S. Asthana, G. Wagner and M. Green for their studies of Rampur, Ramdaua, Viyalo and Umueke respectively.

data, whilst at the same time yielding the benefits of a social anthropological approach. In part this reflected our desire to ask the sorts of questions which an economist would put, but within a structure which facilitated the collection of high quality data.

To this end a number of extensive guidelines and questionnaires were constructed. Although national and international variations were inevitable - and indeed desired - the questionnaires were necessary to ensure at least a minimal degree of cross-cultural standardisation. The basic tool for this purpose was a census form used for the whole of each population, and from which various stratified random samples were drawn. Basic demographic data were recorded, as well as information relating to ethnicity, migration, education, land and livestock ownership, and basic economic activities. Other 100% data were gathered through genealogies. Stratified random samples of 10-15% were taken for the collection of data on household budgets, time allocations, productive and non-productive property, inputs and outputs of major crops, and farming innovations.

In addition to this basic data, three main questionnaires were utilised for the areas of agriculture, migration, and the value of children. The first of these included some thirty sections designed to measure existing and potential innovative tendencies in agriculture. For migration a framework for cross-cultural comparison of the role of migration in absorbing population growth was constructed. This framework provided a solution to the definitional problems inherent in migration studies and included various permutations of categories relating to residence and membership of the societies. A complete quantitative picture of demographic inflows and outflows could thus be built.[7]

The final major questionnaire aimed at providing a socio-economic cost/benefit analysis of children. Whilst such an attempt is self-evidently littered with pitfalls, not the least of which is the impossibility of quantifying certain aspects of the perceived benefits and costs, it was felt that the non-quantitative data gathered throughout the fieldwork period would strengthen the analysis and justify its use. Structured questions on the potential benefits derived from children covered labour inputs (agricultural and wage labour, care of livestock, food preparation, etc.), contribution to flow of income (age of separation from parents, percentage of income used to subsidise family expenditure etc.), and social security (care of aged, kin networks, welfare facilities etc.). Questions relating to costs included household expenditure (opportunity cost of mothers' time, increased food consumption, etc.), education (sex differentials, sibling preference etc.) as well as expenditure on clothing and life cycle rituals, such as dowry,

---

7. Major assistance was provided by Howard Steppler in respect of the agriculture questionnaire, and by Mick Moore for his work on the migration framework.

bridewealth, and birth, marriage and death ceremonies. Additional data were derived from available local and regional official records such as censuses, voters lists, and land registration and sales records.

In summary, data were collected on two levels. At the macro level the broad categories were topography, population, economic characteristics, political structure, religious systems, administrative organisation and infrastructure. At the micro level the above categories were replicated where relevant with a stress on economic characteristics and the cultural system.

Having briefly outlined the methodological and theoretical perspectives of the project, we now turn to a consideration of the substantive issues raised by the research. In Chapter 2 Tim Dyson completes the introduction with an analysis of the project's demographic data. Here the first problem to be confronted concerns the inevitable questions arising out of the interpretation of quantitative data from such relatively small-scale societies: how meaningful are the aggregate statistics? Are cross-cultural generalisations valid? Is the empirical base sufficiently strong to provide genuine results from sophisticated techniques of analysis? After overcoming these hurdles the data is discussed in terms of age/sex distributions, fertility, mortality, and the general implications of population growth.

Part 2 consists of three papers which discuss the interplay between fertility and culture from different standpoints. Joseph Ssennyonga begins by questioning the assumption that a reduction in fertility is a *sine qua non* of higher living standards for the poor: 'observed fertility behaviour has increasingly shown that the poorest tend to be least convinced by the logic of this proposition' (see p. 45), and argues that individuals and collectivities can draw on different cultural inventories in order to respond to new problems and pressures. It is seen to be futile to suggest family limitation to a group whose cultural inventory was formulated long before the increasing man/land ratio created population pressure, particularly in the absence of new options being provided in other aspects of their cultural environment.[8]

Above all two main themes come through clearly as determinants of fertility behaviour; firstly the close inter-dependence between demographic and socio-economic factors, and secondly the observation that those who have the opportunity to control and participate in the processes which govern their lives are more likely to limit their fertility. As a generalised policy proposition there can be no doubt that investment in rural development rather than costly family planning programmes is the key to

8. A documentary film - *Maragoli* - has recently been made in this village by independent film-maker Sandy Nichols with the author's consultation.

balanced local and regional growth. Put another way - as suggested at Bucharest - look after the people and population will take care of itself.

The impact of culture and ethnicity on fertility behaviour is further examined in Sammy Onwuazor's discussion of abortion and family size in Umueke, a Nigerian village. Using the extended case study method, Onwuazor analyses the normative pressures surrounding the actors in an alleged case of unlawful carnal knowledge and abortion, and the subsequent repercussions within the village when the formalistic procedures of modern law clash with the traditional methods of solving such disputes.

The high incidence of abortion in the village is at least partially explained by the fact that the women of the village were hardly aware of any other means of family planning. Whilst there was a tacit agreement at the Bucharest Conference not to raise the subject of abortion (although there was some discussion in the contemporaneous Population Tribune), our studies suggest that - where culturally viable - and certainly as an interim measure - greater efforts should be made to provide safe and effective abortion facilities.

Part 2 concludes with an examination by Monica Das Gupta of the actual mechanisms of fertility change in a north Indian village, previously studied by Oscar Lewis in 1953. A discussion of macro perspectives such as demographic transition theory and micro approaches like cost/benefit analyses finds both lacking. The former is felt to be inadequate because such variables as education and modernisation are considered on an abstract level, and the latter is rejected as being too highly individual oriented. An alternative model is proposed which stresses the mediating influence of group norms on the relationship between the economic environment on the one hand, and individual fertility behaviour on the other. The analytical gap between macro and micro perspectives is bridged by concentrating on the mechanisms through which fertility behaviour is influenced.

The third part of this study moves to a closer consideration of the interaction between economic forces and population growth. Mukul Dube spent much time not only living in a North Indian village characterised by high rates of intra-rural migration, he also lived and travelled with various migrant groups in their search for work throughout the region. In contrast to Rampur, the village discussed in Chapter 5 by Das Gupta, many other villages in India, such as this one, are unable to meet their peak labour requirements.

It is important to stress that whilst population pressure is a contributory factor to this phenomenon, the solution is to be found not in stepping up investment in costly family planning programmes, or even in the recent measures of compulsory sterilisation introduced in parts of India - a strategy which is probably doomed to failure in any event - but rather in the provision of employment and educational opportunities within a framework of wider socio-economic development.

These themes are echoed in Newton Gunasinghe's study of a Kandyan village in Sri Lanka. Here Gunasinghe argues that the observed fertility decline in recent years is attributable to various factors generally associated with economic development, but which in fact he sees as being part of a much wider process of under-development. Drawing on the centre-periphery model within a dependency theory framework, the work of Baran and Frank is cited to show that the integration of the village he studied into the national economy has created a situation whereby development consists of a process of resource transfer along a similar path, with the fruits of economic expansion going ultimately to the international commercial metropolises. This process is replicated at the international level with resource transfer to the metropolitan centres. The development of the rural infrastructure is not seen as genuine economic development, but rather as the establishment of the minimal conditions which will facilitate this flow of resources from rural to urban centres. This uneven development process results in accumulation in the metropolis and stagnation in the hinterlands. It is this process and not the postulations of demographic transition theory which account for the declining rate of fertility in Sri Lanka. It is apparent that despite the radically different ideological base of this argument and the conceptual framework used, many of the features observed are similar in nature to those documented in the previous and ensuing chapters of this study.

It should be stressed here that education and health services, the communication network and the transport system, have all been developed in Sri Lanka to a greater extent than in most of the Indian and African areas under consideration. Nonetheless this expansion is still basically service-oriented, so that the benefits are being channelled away from the rural areas to the national and ultimately international commercial centres. This situation - of declining fertility on the one hand and rural under development on the other - highlights the fallibility of a purely family planning approach to population issues. If even the perpetuation of underdevelopment can bring about fertility declines, we are surely forced to reconsider the alleged benefits of such declines and consequently also the policies which attempt to bring them about at the expense of the poor themselves.

The second Sri Lankan study takes a different perspective. By concentrating on the micro-level mechanisms which bring about changes in fertility behaviour, the author shows that different household decision-making models are required to understand attitudes to family size amongst groups in different socio-economic strata.

Against a similar background of declining mortality and fertility rates W.M. Tilakaratne shows that the principal causes of declining fertility in his village are also to be found in the rising age at marriage and reduced marital fertility. These latter factors in turn reflect changes in the socio-economic structure and the increased provision of welfare facilities. It is precisely the delineation of these changes at the micro level which increase our knowledge of the impact of 'modernising' variables on household decision-making processes.

The overall picture exhibits broad similarities to the first Sri Lankan study. The provision of education and health services has increased the villagers' perception of the options open to them, and this, together with the provision of limited employment opportunities, has played a prominent part in reducing fertility. However, the positive correlation between lack of education and high fertility clearly illustrates that those who remain in an agrarian sector whose general development is neglected within the wider economy have a constant incentive to produce large numbers of children.

The fourth paper in this section stresses the interplay between education, poverty and fertility amongst the Wataita tribe of Southern Kenya. Despite the evident differences between this area and the two Sri Lankan villages, the factors which influence fertility decisions display a remarkable similarity. Against the backcloth of an extremely high national population growth rate (3.3% p.a.), it is seen that one facet of the first stage of economic development which is widespread in Africa - the individualisation and consolidation of land ownership in societies where land was hitherto communally owned and worked - has brought with it a dependence on non-agricultural work which is not generally available.

Policy recommendations arising from the study suggest the need for breaking down the self-perpetuating syndrome of poverty, rapid population growth and differential access to education. The use of non-labour displacing intermediate technologies would increase productivity within the agrarian sector and reduce the dependence on the limited number of employment opportunities available elsewhere. For those who already have the incentive to limit fertility it is suggested that family planning programmes be more closely integrated in the overall strategy of rural development. Drawing on the lessons learned from the Chinese experience discussed in the penultimate chapter, an effective way of ensuring that the demands produced by a growing population do not outstrip available local resources would be the communalisation of decisions relating to family size and resource production. Such an approach would certainly be more consistent with earlier social structures than the present tendency towards individualisation, and this type of cultural continuity could well provide the basis for collective prosperity and help narrow the increasing gap between rich and poor.

For the final paper in this section we return to India. Vinod Jairath's analysis of village Ramdaua shows a co-existence of two phenomena: the highest mortality rates of all the villages studied (28% Infant Mortality Rate), and the highest fertility. By any socio-economic indicators this village is at an extremely primitive stage of general development. One of the most common observations in the village is 'rich farmers invest in tractors, the poor invest in children'. The introduction of modern technologies has resulted in a declining demand for labour, and since the district as a whole is relatively under-developed alternative employment possibilities are limited. It remains to be seen whether or not the realisation of these diminishing employment prospects will result in conscious limitation of family size.

The prospect of medical technology reducing mortality rates in the near future necessitates a rapid improvement in family planning education, and at the same time the provision of serious measures to counter the growing inequalities. With a low population growth rate, and a growing recognition of the high costs involved in child-rearing and bearing, it is evident that the problem is not population, but rather the fate of those people who have yet to benefit from the fruits of a development pattern which exhibits such inequalities.

The final section of this study deals with the policy and planning implications of various approaches to population issues. The first part summarises the lessons to be learnt from the Chinese experience, and although Penny Kane is not a member of the main research team we were nonetheless pleased to have the benefit of her personal experience in China. This adds an important dimension to our perspectives, not least because the success of Chinese economic development has always been something of an enigma to Western observers, and this success appears to have continued in the field of balanced population growth. If the world's most populous - and still mainly agrarian-based - country can reduce its birthrate within the space of five years from 32 to 19 per 1000, there are inevitably policy implications for Third World planners, even those operating in a radically different ideological context.

The Chinese experience seems to have created a situation whose two principle components appear to be vital in bringing about voluntary family size limitation. The first of these is the provision of genuine social security - including old age security, which is generally found to be a significant factor in influencing desired number of children. The second is the extent to which individuals feel able to control their socio-economic environment. When people are convinced that individual decisions and choices have a public impact, and when they feel that their role in the social, economic and political systems is significant, they are more likely to ensure that the nature of their own fertility decisions is in harmony with the needs of the wider socio-economic system.

Both of these themes are taken up in Scarlett Epstein's overall synthesis of the project's data and hypotheses. Stressing the importance of analysing fertility behaviour in the context of all the other determining variables, and not as an isolated or exogenous factor as has hitherto been the case, it is argued that a demographic transition in Third World countries cannot be expected until the people are in a position to exert a positive influence on their own and their children's socio-physical environment. Thus 'a radical restructuring of social systems seems to be a necessary pre-condition of successful fertility control' (see p.221). Two models are then developed which delineate the inter-relationships between variables such as education, level of technology, mortality and fertility, different combinations of which produce either an 'accommodating' or an 'intervening' relationship with the socio-physical environment.

The former approach is prevalent in closed societies characterised by high fertility and morbidity rates, primitive technology, labour intensive agrarian methods and general conditions of extreme uncertainty which render planning virtually impossible. In such societies it is not cost/benefit considerations which determine family size, but rather adaptation to a hostile environment in which children are considered essential for the very survival of the society. Accommodation is manifested in attitudes to fertility mentioned earlier, for example that children are born because of Karma, fate or God's will.

These societies then undergo a transitionary phase in which modernising influences occur. The introduction of medical facilities decreases mortality rates and creates population pressure. Gradually the spread of education and agricultural technology leads to more certainty and control over the environment, albeit by the elite rather than the majority. This process changes people's aspirations and initiates consideration for the quality of their own and their children's lives, culminating in fertility reduction.

Results of the study show that the introduction of education and new technologies involves a better harnessing of available resources and hence a better life. But differential access to these aspects of modernisation causes structural inequalities, and accounts for different fertility behaviour amongst different sections of the population. Those who do enter the upward spiral develop an interventive approach; continued poverty for those who do not - and whose poverty may even increase - results in unchanged attitudes to their socio-physical environment which is reflected in unchanged fertility behaviour. Turning to policy suggestions for family planning programmes, the observation that family planning only works for those who want it is reiterated. The vast mass who remain untouched by modernising influences evidently do not. Similarly, most contraceptives currently recommended are pre-conception methods, which demand a degree of planning that cannot be expected in a world which is perceived as being shaped by forces beyond people's control. Post-conception methods of family limitation have been largely ignored, although abortion has existed in every society since time immemorial. In terms of cultural complementarity the legalisation of abortion, the development of abortive pills and research into traditional contraceptive methods may prove to be a more viable and effective strategy than continued high investment in Western contraceptive technology. Most important of all, however, is the need to change the socio-economic environments which ultimately shape people's attitudes to fertility. Provision of the means of limiting family size must always be a secondary consideration as long as the incentive to do so is lacking.

Global annual increases in population have fallen from 69 million in 1970 to 64 million in 1975. It is estimated that although the acceptance of modern family planning methods has played a significant role in bringing about this fall, the declining growth rates in the Third World can be attributed to increased mortality rates due to malnutrition and starvation. With the prospect of declining international aid and comparative current stagnation in Western capitalist societies, the outlook for the rural poor is bleak. Planners and academics alike must realise that now - perhaps more than ever before - the emphasis must lie on rural development rather than investment in costly family planning programmes, whose influence in these areas is of doubtful value unless complemented by strategies which ensure that the living conditions of Third World people and their children are raised sufficiently from the depths of poverty to enable them to survive today, let alone plan for tomorrow.

CHAPTER 2

AN ANALYSIS OF VILLAGE FERTILITY, MORTALITY AND GROWTH[1]

INTRODUCTION

Anthropologists have become more interested recently in demographic issues. However despite this growing interest, relatively few studies by social anthropologists have attempted to take specific account of demographic factors. In part this is because it has not always been practical to apply demographic techniques to communities of the size often studied. But another reason is a general lack of interest in collecting and presenting quantitative data (see, e.g. Nag 1962).

A prime concern of the study currently under way at the Institute of Development Studies is the relationship between rural poverty and population growth. The focus of this chapter is population growth, and its main purpose is to present some reasonably reliable information on both the relative rates and components (i.e. fertility, mortality and migration) of population growth in the project villages.[2]

The analysis makes direct use of only two sets of information: the age-sex distribution of each village population, and the response of women aged 15 and over to questions on the number of live births ever born to them, and the number of these infants reported at the interview as having subsequently died. With reference to the questions on births and deaths it is worth noting that they are 'retrospective' - this greatly increases the number of vital events 'caught' by the interviewer. Moreover, both the form and sequence of the questions was specifically designed to obviate the difficulties commonly encountered in questioning.

---

1. This is an amended version of a paper presented at the Conference on 'A Cross-cultural Study of Population Growth and Rural Poverty' held at the Institute of Development Studies in December 1975. The author wishes to stress that the paper presents an analysis of *preliminary* findings. As more data is processed so other types of analysis will become possible and the picture outlined here should be confirmed and refined. The author wishes to thank the members of the IDS Population Project for making available the raw demographic data for each village, and Scarlett Epstein, John Simons and Michael Teitelbaum for helpful suggestions.
2. The village of Mulkipur, studied by Mukul Dube, has been excluded, since the relevant demographic data was collected during a subsequent field visit and has not yet been analysed.

TABLE 2.1

Age distributions* and sex ratios by broad age groups

VILLAGE:	BOGAMUWA			DELUMGODA			UMUEKE			RAMDAUA			RAMPUR			VIYALO			TAITA		
Age group	Males	Females	SR	Males	Females	SR	Males	Females	SR	Males	Females	SR	Males	Females	SR	Males	Females	SR	Males	Females	SR
0– 4	58 (7.04)	85 (9.64)	68	32 (9.64)	32 (9.12)	100	33 (20.25)	31 (16.06)	106	97 (15.18)	77 (14.50)	126	169 (15.93)	133 (14.60)	127	165 (22.12)	156 (19.19)	106	204 (16.52)	239 (17.62)	85
5–14	202 (24.51)	222 (25.17)	91	75 (22.59)	93 (26.50)	81	56 (34.35)	35 (18.13)	160	174 (27.23)	140 (26.37)	124	279 (26.30)	254 (27.88)	110	248 (33.24)	256 (31.49)	97	371 (30.04)	394 (29.03)	94
15–44	383 (46.48)	412 (46.71)	93	166 (50.00)	167 (47.57)	99	48 (29.45)	95 (49.23)	31	260 (40.69)	228 (42.93)	114	445 (41.94)	403 (44.24)	110	225 (30.16)	293 (36.04)	77	498 (40.32)	569 (41.93)	88
45+	181 (21.97)	163 (18.48)	111	59 (17.77)	59 (16.81)	100	26 (15.95)	32 (16.58)	81	108 (16.90)	86 (16.20)	88	168 (15.83)	121 (13.28)	139	108 (14.48)	108 (13.28)	100	162 (13.12)	155 (11.42)	105
Total	824 (100.00)	882 (100.00)	93	332 (100.00)	351 (100.00)	95	163 (100.00)	193 (100.00)	84	639 (100.00)	531 (100.00)	120	1061 (100.00)	911 (100.00)	116	746 (100.00)	813 (100.00)	92	1235 (100.00)	1357 (100.00)	91

* The percentage age-distributions are given in brackets.

The raw data collected will be shown to be meaningful in itself - before translation into more conventional demographic measures.[3]

The present analysis will make use of demographic 'model' distributions. Working usually on populations larger than those under discussion here, demographers have assembled a body of hypothetical 'models' which broadly represent basic demographic structures and processes. These models, which are usually based on some averaging of empirical observations, are not always systematized under the rubric of 'model'. They range in complexity from interval scales of population growth to mathematical constructs representing mortality. In this paper, the type of model used is known as a model life table: a specification of the mortality experience of a hypothetical population. The main assumption underlying the use of models for purposes such as those in this chapter, is that over the long run, small-scale populations are subject to processes and constraints similar to those of larger groups.

Finally it should be stated that any demographic analysis of a 'developing' society is confronted by many possible pitfalls. Moreover the smaller the population, the harder it is to gauge the underlying levels of fertility and mortality. Therefore there can be nothing sacrosanct about the estimates reported in this paper. They will need to be cross-checked against other types of data, as well as against sources more usually collected by anthropologists (e.g. genealogies). In other words the estimates need to be shown to be consistent with other findings. However, it is a contention of this paper that meaningful - if approximate - estimates of demographic parameters can be obtained in the typical anthropological fieldwork situation, and in particular that retrospective questioning, employed in conjunction with model distributions, can greatly extend the range of anthropological demographic studies.[4]

The Age/Sex Distributions

Table 2.1 gives the age/sex distributions of the project villages by broad age-groups (0-4, 5-14, 15-44, and 45+). It is possible to discern several interesting features from these distributions. To begin with, in all but the two Indian villages (Rampur and Ramdaua) the overall sex ratio (males per hundred females) is below 100. The ratio is particularly low in Umueke, although

---

3. For the use of these questions and the associated techniques see for example, Brass, W., *et al*, *The Demography of Tropical Africa*, Princeton; Princeton University Press, 1968, and, United Nations, *Manual IV - Methods of Estimating Basic Demographic Measures for Incomplete Data*, (Population Studies No. 42), New York, 1967.
4. For a further discussion of possible methodological strategies in this form of enquiry see Dyson, T., *On The Relationship Between Demography and Social Anthropology*, IDS Discussion Paper No. 68, Institute of Development Studies 1975.

it should be noted that this village is numerically very small. Although these low sex ratios could all in part reflect higher mortality of males (sex differentials in mortality have not yet been analyzed), they might also be due to differential out-migration of males. In all villages except Rampur and Ramdaua, the sex ratio for the age-group 15-44 is below 100 - although it is only slightly less so in Delumgoda and Bogamuwa. However the particularly low ratios at 15-44 in Viyalo and Umueke suggest differential out-migration of males at these ages. Onwuazor's more detailed analysis of data on both the resident and non-resident population of Umueke confirms this suggestion. The overall sex ratio of the former is 84 while the sex ratio of the non-resident population is 142.[5]

Several interesting points arise from the percentage age-distribution by sex that are also given in Table 2.1. Perhaps the single most informative feature is the differential percentage distribution at age-group 0-4. In Delumgoda and Bogamuwa only around 9% of the total population is aged 0-4. The corresponding figures for the remaining five villages are much higher - ranging from 14% to 22% of the total. Although there could be a number of reasons behind such differences, taken together they imply that fertility is probably relatively low in the two Sri Lankan communities. We should note also the comparatively large percentages of the population at ages 45 and over, in both Delumgoda and Bogamuwa. In the latter over 20% of the total population fall into this open-ended age-group. In general we can say that these two age-distributions show that these populations are distinctly older than the other five - and again this is particularly true for Bogamuwa.

Table 2.2 gives dependency ratios - i.e. ratios that express estimates of the numbers of young and old as a percentage of those 'economically active' (here defined as those aged between 15 and 64) - for all seven villages. Clearly this index is arbitrary in the definition of both 'dependent' and 'economically active'. However, it remains useful as a characterizing measure of the total population, and can usefully add to the

5. See Chapter 4, p. 86. Males migrate out while in the more economically active age-groups, but return to the village at later ages. Onwuazor quotes Uchendu as saying "Almost from the start the individual is aware of his dependence on his kin groups and his community ... it is his ultimate desire to return to his village after earning money elsewhere. To him, the village is the appropriate place for retirement, the city a place to earn money". This return migration also occurs in Viyalo: see Chapter 3, p. 63.

TABLE 2.2

Dependency ratios

Village	Dependency ratio*
Bogamuwa	62
Delumgoda	65
Umueke	96
Ramdaua	82
Rampur	83
Viyalo	135
Taita	96

* Persons of 'dependent' ages (i.e. 0-14 and 65+) per 100 persons of 'working' ages (i.e. 15-64).

TABLE 2.3

Child/woman ratios

Village	CWR* (0-4)	CWR** (0-14)
Bogamuwa	0.35	1.38
Delumgoda	0.38	1.39
Umueke	0.65	1.72
Ramdaua	0.76	2.14
Rampur	0.75	2.07
Viyalo	1.10	2.82
Taita	0.78	2.12

* The ratio of the population aged 0-4 to the number of women aged 15-44.

** The ratio of the population aged 0-14 to the number of women aged 15-44.

interpretation of the age/sex distributions. Again Table 2.2 suggests that Delumgoda and Bogamuwa are demographically different from the remaining five villages, since in both the dependency ratio is comparatively low.[6] The ratios are high for Ramdaua and Rampur (82/83) and also for Taita and Umueke (96). Viyalo has by far the greatest dependency burden (135) - a ratio over twice as high as those for Delumgoda and Bogamuwa. Although the age-groups used in Table 2.1 are not exactly comparable with those used to calculate the dependency ratios, it can be seen that of all the villages Viyalo has by far the smallest percentage (33%) of its population aged 15-44. Even Umueke, with heavy male out-migration, has 40% of its population between ages 15 and 44. While Viyalo's sex ratio at 15-44 suggests differential out-migration of males at these ages, the percentage breakdowns give some indication that females aged 15-44 have also out-migrated from Viyalo.

Table 2.3 gives two sets of child/adult ratios (CAR's) - a simple index of fertility - computed for each of the seven village populations. It can be variously defined, but here the child/adult ratio refers to the ratio of children aged 0-4 (and 0-14), to women aged 15-44 years. Fortunately both these components of the population are usually relatively unaffected by migration. Plainly the index is imperfect as a measure of fertility, in that it is affected by mortality and possibly migration. However it can be computed for the village situations for which data for ordinary birth rates is often unavailable. The child/adult ratios suggest much the same village fertility ranking whichever ratio (0-4 or 0-14) is chosen. Table 2.3 suggests that fertility is lowest in Bogamuwa. Delumgoda also seems to have relatively low fertility. Umueke's child/adult ratios suggest substantially higher fertility. The child/adult ratios for Rampur, Ramdaua and Taita suggest high and broadly comparable levels of fertility. Finally, Viyalo has by far the highest child/adult ratios; however we have seen that there is evidence of out-migration of adult females from this village, and this may well have distorted the child/adult ratio upwards.

Fertility

We can get a better idea of the relative fertility levels of the villages by examining the mean number of live births ever born per woman. These mean parity values are given in Table 2.4 for five year age-groups of women from 15-19 up to 45-49. The mean parity of all women aged 40-49 is also presented. Less reliance can be put on the parity values for women aged 15-19 and 20-24 as they are based on relatively few live births. However, for almost all age-groups of women, the reported parities

---

6. For purposes of comparison here are some dependency ratios for some national populations: Philippines (1948): 90, Mexico (1950): 82, India (1951): 71, France (1954): 55, and United States (1950): 55. These ratios are taken from Barclay, G., *Techniques of Population Analysis*, Wiley, New York, 1958 p. 267.

TABLE 2.4

Parity ratios for women aged 15-49

Village	Age Group of Women							Mean Parity of Women
	15-19	20-24	25-29	30-34	35-39	40-44	45-49	40-49
Bogamuwa	0.03	0.45	1.07	2.32	3.48	3.95	3.30	3.60
Delumgoda	0.00	0.15	1.58	2.57	3.95	6.38	6.61	6.49
Umueke	0.48	0.58	2.17	4.00	4.54	6.25	5.67	6.15
Ramdaua	0.46	2.07	4.08	6.48	7.79	7.21	8.12	7.75
Rampur	0.09	1.70	3.61	5.27	6.36	6.40	7.17	7.05
Viyalo	0.15	1.28	3.17	5.96	8.88	8.18	9.53	8.58
Taita	1.27	2.41	4.40	5.96	7.15	7.93	7.96	7.94

agree with the child/adult ratios in suggesting that fertility is lowest in Bogamuwa. Not only is fertility currently low in Bogamuwa, but the ratios also suggest that it has been relatively low for some period of time. Thus women at the very end of their reproductive cycle, aged 40-49, have had on average only 3.6 live births per woman - this is about half the level of the same index for the other villages. The fact that fertility is relatively low, and that it has apparently been so for a considerable period of time (15-20 years), is entirely consistent with, and in large part probably explains, the aforementioned fact that Bogamuwa has the oldest age-structure of all the villages. In fact the detailed Bogamuwa age-structure shows that the 5-9 age-group is considerably smaller than that at 10-14, and in turn the age-group 0-4 is markedly smaller than that at 5-9. Although fertility has always been relatively low in Bogamuwa, it may nevertheless have fallen still further over the past few years.[7]

The other Sri Lankan village, Delumgoda, is much smaller, and any conclusions must therefore be put forward more tentatively in this case. However, for all age-groups of women up to 35-39, Delumgoda has the second lowest mean parity values. The fertility experience of these women (aged 15-39), as expressed by the parity values, is therefore consistent with the suggestion of the child/adult ratios, namely that over the recent past Delumgoda has had the second lowest level of fertility. Again the detailed age-structure shows that the numbers at 5-9 are smaller than those at 10-14, and again the numbers at 0-4 fall well below those at 5-9. However, at later ages, women in Delumgoda have borne over twice as many live births on average as women in Bogamuwa. The parity ratios at 40-44 and 45-49 are high (6.4 and 6.6 live births respectively) - in fact they are above the corresponding parities for women in Umueke. The general conclusion to be drawn is that Delumgoda has reduced its fertility from previously high levels.[8]

The mean parity values in Table 2.4 support the indications of the child/adult ratios, that the village with the third lowest level of fertility is Umueke. There is no easily discernible suggestion of any recent fertility decline. However overall the parity values are perhaps not as high as one might expect: on average women aged 40-49 have had just over six live births. Today the resident population of Umueke is actually smaller than when the village was first surveyed in 1937. It is at least possible that over this period (1937-74) male out-migration has had a depressing effect on fertility.

The mean parities for Rampur at age-groups 30-34, 35-39, 40-44 and 45-49, fall well below those of the remaining three villages. Again, the general indications of the child/adult

---

7. For additional evidence suggesting that this is probably the case see Tilakaratne's analysis, Chapter 8.
8. This fertility decline is confirmed and analyzed by Newton Gunasinghe: see Chapter 7.

TABLE 2.5

Fertility indices

Village	Mean Number of Live Births per Women Aged 15-49	Standardized Mean* No. of live Births per Women Aged 15-49	Mean Parity of Women Aged 40-49	Crude Birth Rate (CBR) Per Thousand Population
Bogamuwa	1.72	1.57	3.60	27.8
Delumgoda	2.12	2.18	6.49	-
Umueke	3.02	2.61	6.15	-
Ramdaua	4.25	4.12	7.75	56.6
Rampur	3.46	3.43	7.05	45.1
Viyalo	4.01	4.01	8.58	49.4
Taita	4.05	4.38	7.94	50.9

* Standardized on the combined age-distribution of women aged 15-19 ... 45-49 in all seven villages.

TABLE 2.6

Proportion of live births now dead, by age-group of women aged 15-49

Village	Age group of women							Proportion Dead, All Ages
	15-19	20-24	25-29	30-34	35-39	40-44	45-49	15-49
Bogamuwa	0.00	0.08	0.05	0.05	0.06	0.07	0.06	0.06
Delumgoda	-	0.00	0.10	0.17	0.10	0.11	0.07	0.10
Umueke	0.00	0.00	0.11	0.27	0.37	0.25	0.35	0.27
Ramdaua	0.35	0.27	0.39	0.46	0.43	0.47	0.51	0.44
Rampur	0.10	0.10	0.18	0.20	0.24	0.22	0.31	0.22
Viyalo	0.09	0.08	0.12	0.14	0.19	0.22	0.33	0.21
Taita	0.07	0.13	0.13	0.12	0.15	0.17	0.26	0.15

ratios as to the relative levels of village fertility seem to be confirmed. However, comparison of the ratios for the remaining three villages is somewhat more problematic. The parity ratios for Ramdaua and Taita suggest that even relatively young women, aged 25-29, have experienced an average of four live births per woman.[9] It can certainly be said that fertility is very high in each of these villages. However the completed fertility of women in all age-groups over 35 is highest in Viyalo - the mean parity of women aged 40-49 is reported to be 8.6 live births.

Two additional fertility ratios have been computed and are given in Table 2.5. The first is the mean number of live births born to all women aged 15-49. The second refers to the same age-group of women (15-49), however in this case the respective parity values for each village have been standardized on a common age-distribution: that of all women aged 15-19 ... 45-49 in all of the villages.[10] As can be seen, both the standardized and unstandardized mean parity values again suggest that fertility is lowest in Bogamuwa, followed by Delumgoda and Umueke. Table 2.5 also implies that Rampur has slightly lower fertility than the remaining three villages.

Mortality

Table 2.6 presents for each age-group of women (15-19 ... 45-49) and for all women combined (ages 15-49), the proportion of their live births which were reported to have subsequently died. Despite smallness of numbers (which probably accounts for much of the fluctuation at young ages, especially in the low-mortality villages), there can be little doubt that infant and childhood mortality is lowest in Bogamuwa. At every age-group women in this village have lost proportionately fewer children than women in any of the other six villages. The village with the next lowest level of mortality is Delumgoda - where women have lost on average 10% of everborn live births, compared with only 6% in Bogamuwa. Women in Taita have lost on average 15% of live births, while in the other Kenyan community, Viyalo, 21% of all children born were reported as having died. In Rampur and Umueke the figures were 22% and 27% respectively. Finally we should note the staggeringly high proportion reported as dead by women in Ramdaua: 44% of all live births to women aged 15-49 were dead at the time the village was surveyed. As can be seen

---

9. Age shifting may be one factor behind these very high parity rates at relatively young ages. In particular the parity of 1.27 for women aged 15-19 in Taita cannot be accepted at face value.
10. This composite age-distribution was chosen because it is in a sense 'neutral'. However choice of a different distribution is unlikely to radically alter the relative ranking of the villages *vis a vis* fertility. The same general comment also applies to the standardization of the 'proportions dead' (see Table 2.7).

TABLE 2.7

Mortality indices

Village	Proportion of live births dead to women aged 15-49	Proportion of* live births dead to women aged 15-49 (standardized)	Expectation of Life at Birth (Years)	Crude Death Rate (per thousand)
Bogamuwa	0.06	0.06	66	8.7
Delumgoda	0.10	0.09	-	-
Umueke	0.27	0.24	-	-
Ramdaua	0.44	0.43	27	37.1
Rampur	0.22	0.21	44	19.9
Viyalo	0.21	0.19	48	14.2
Taita	0.15	0.16	52	13.9

* Standardized on the combined age-distribution of live births ever born to women aged 15-19 to 45-49, in all villages

TABLE 2.8

Measures of population growth

Village	Mean No. of live Births Surviving per Woman (15-49)	Mean No. of live Births Surviving per Woman, Standardized (15-49)	Crude Rate of Natural Increase (% per year)
Bogamuwa	1.62	1.48	1.9
Delumgoda	1.90	1.97	-
Umueke	2.20	1.98	-
Ramdaua	2.40	2.33	1.9
Rampur	2.70	2.70	2.5
Viyalo	3.18	3.25	3.5
Taita	3.45	3.67	3.7

in Ramdaua (Table 2.6), women of all ages reported an exceedingly high child mortality loss.

Table 2.7 gives the corresponding standardized proportion of live births now dead - (standardized on the combined age-distribution of all live births to women aged 15-49 in all the villages). It can be seen that standardization by age makes relatively little difference to both the overall and comparative levels of mortality in each of the villages.

Population Growth

Having examined the levels of fertility, mortality, (and to a lesser extent migration) in each of the villages, we can now approach the problem of determining their comparative standing in terms of population growth.

Table 2.8 gives two indices of growth that can be readily computed from the basic measures examined so far. The first is the mean number of live births surviving to all women aged 15-59; this is the product of the mean number of live births born to all women aged 15-49, and secondly the reciprocal of the proportion of all live births that were reported as dead. The second measure that can be computed is the age-standardized equivalent of the first i.e. the standardized number of live births surviving to all women aged 15-49. Because these two measures have both fertility and mortality components, they can be taken as indicators of natural rates of population growth. However it must be noted they represent the experience of women at all ages (15-49). This has the advantage that the measures are based on larger numbers, but the drawback that women of different ages may not have experienced exactly the same fertility or mortality levels.[11]

Both measures of the average number of live births surviving per woman, give roughly the same picture as to the rates of natural population growth in the seven communities.

Let us first examine the unstandardized measures. Bogamuwa has the lowest average number of live births surviving per woman; perhaps this is not surprising in view of its comparatively low fertility levels extending back over a considerable period of time. But it is worth remembering that Bogamuwa also has the lowest levels of mortality. The figures suggest that the two East African communities (particularly Taita), with very high levels of fertility and relatively low levels of mortality, are growing the fastest. In both of them an average of over three children are surviving to women aged 15-49 years. Although Ramdaua also shares very high levels of fertility, the mean number of children actually surviving to women in this village is

---

11. For example a recent decline in age-specific fertility rates at young ages would be obscured because the measure aggregates the experience of younger and older women.

markedly lower than in Taita or Viyalo. This is due to the very high mortality levels prevailing in Ramdaua.

As stated previously, the age-standardized rates give a very similar picture. The only exception is Umueke, where the mean number of children surviving per woman is slightly reduced. The standardized rates suggest that the number of children surviving in this village is comparable with that in Delumgoda. The issue is difficult to resolve, especially in view of the small numbers on which the relevant ratios are based - particularly in Umueke. However it is clear that standardization reduced both fertility and mortality measures in Umueke, whilst not appreciably affecting those in Delumgoda. This is partly because over the relevant age-range (15-49) the female age-structure of the Nigerian village is actually older than that in Delumgoda. The reduction in the mean number of live births ever born to women aged 45-49, resulting from the standardization, coupled with the still heavy mortality measures, is enough to reduce the standardized mean number of children surviving to a figure comparable with that in Delumgoda. Apart from this, however, we have seen that the age-progression of parity values in Delumgoda indicates that there has been a decline in fertility over the last two decades. As mentioned earlier, the measures currently under discussion aggregate the fertility experience of women at all ages and stages of the reproductive cycle. In view of this recent fertility decline in Delumgoda, it may well be that its population is currently growing at a slower rate than that of Umueke. The mean numbers of children surviving to women at younger ages would support this view.[12]

Further Analysis

So far the computation and analysis have utilized relatively basic information. Nevertheless, we have been able to obtain a definite idea as to the relative standing of each of the villages as regards fertility, mortality and natural increase. In the following paragraphs an attempt is made where possible to translate these measures into rough estimates of more conventional demographic indices.[13] However it must be emphasized that the

---

12. The mean numbers of children surviving to women by age-group in the two villages are:

Age Group of Women:	20-24	25-29	30-34	35-39	40-44	45-49
Delumgoda	0.151	1.419	2.144	3.573	5.695	6.115
Umueke	0.583	1.917	2.900	2.850	4.665	3.672

13. The small numbers in Delumgoda and Umueke prohibited the additional analysis of data in these two villages.

following estimates are very approximate, and they must be considered provisional in that they do not incorporate any analysis of additional data collected.[14]

On the assumption of constant fertility, the mean parity of women at the end of the reproductive cycle would equal the total fertility rate prevailing in the community. In fact experience suggests that the reported mean parity of women aged 45-49 is usually an underestimate of total fertility, owing to a variety of 'memory errors'. It seems reasonable to assume, both from the reported parity values and the ethnographic accounts, that there has been little if any fertility decline in Taita, Viyalo, Rampur and Ramdaua - though this is not true for Bogamuwa and Delumgoda. Moreover the in-depth interviewing and cross-checking by fieldworkers should have minimized memory errors insofar as was possible. The procedure adopted here is therefore to take the mean parity of women aged 40-49 as a rough measure of total fertility. This parity value may still represent a slight underestimate of the TFR, if for no other reason than that a few women aged 40-49 will give birth before they become infecund. However, use of the measure draws some support from the very high mean parity values that were in fact reported. It is certainly unlikely that these parity values overstate the level of total fertility.[15]

General indications as to the overall level of mortality, expressed in terms of life expectation, were obtained from the proportions of live births reported as dead for all villages except Umueke and Delumgoda. These proportions were converted into

---

14. Additional data collected includes for example information on parent-survivorship.

15. The original intention was to 'mark-up' by a reasonable percentage (say 10%) the parity of women aged 45-49, in order to get an estimate of the total fertility rate (TFR). However, a rule of thumb that may have some purpose when dealing with data collected as part of a large census, is not necessarily applicable in a situation of intensive local-level study. The fieldworkers were well-versed in the various biases and kinds of 'memory error' associated with this question on ever-born live births. They were thus in a situation to minimize such response errors. Therefore it seems better to accept the parity values of older women at face value. The responses of women in age-groups 40-44 and 45-49 were averaged to produce a slightly more reliable figure based on larger numbers. Nevertheless, for reasons stated earlier, this parity value (40-49) may be a slight underestimate of the TFR. In this connection, however, it is worth drawing attention to how high the reported mean parity values are at later ages, and also to the absence in most of the villages, of a 'fall-off' in the parity values at later ages, which would indicate failure to 'pick up' some of the live births borne to older women.

TABLE 2.9

Mortality levels (expressed in terms of life expectation) corresponding to the proportions of live births now dead, by age group of women (see also Table 2.6)

Village	Age group of women						
	15-19	20-24	25-29	30-34	35-39	40-44	45-49
Bogamuwa	-	52.5-55.0	63.2-65.8	65.8-68.2	65.8-68.2	65.8-68.2	68.2-70.2
Ramdaua	22.5-25.0	32.5-35.0	25.0-27.5	22.5-25.0	27.5-30.0	27.5-30.0	27.5-30.0
Rampur	45.0-47.5	50.0-52.5	42.5-45.0	45.0-47.5	42.5-45.0	47.5-50.0	42.5-45.0
Viyalo	45.0-47.5	55.0-57.6	50.0-52.5	50.0-52.5	47.5-50.0	45.0-47.5	37.5-40.0
Taita	47.5-50.0	45.0-47.5	50.0-52.5	55.0-57.6	52.5-55.0	52.5-55.0	45.0-47.5

life-table (lx) values using a technique developed by Brass.[16] The resulting life-table functions were 'matched' against life tables of varying life-expectancies in a standard model system.[17] The range of life expectations implied by the various values of 'proportions dead' for different age-groups of respondents are given in Table 2.9. Again, less reliance can be put on the values stemming from the replies of women aged 15-19 and 20-24, as they are based on only a few live births, and even fewer deaths. Nevertheless it should be stressed that the implied range of values of life-expectation resulting from the responses of women aged 25 to 44 are reasonably consistent. They can be summarized as follows:-

Village	Life expectation at birth (years)		
	lower bound	upper bound	range[18]
Bogamuwa	63.2	68.2	5.0
Ramdaua	22.5	30.0	7.5
Rampur	42.5	50.0	7.5
Viyalo	45.0	52.5	7.5
Taita	50.0	57.6	7.6

The response of women aged 25-29, 30-34, 35-39 and 40-44, when converted into life-table functions, correspond to l_3 l_5 l_{10} and l_{15} respectively, i.e. their response can be taken to refer to some average of the mortality experience of the previous fifteen years or so. For each of the remaining five villages (i.e. Bogamuwa, Ramdaua, Rampur, Viyalo and Taita) these four lx values were averaged together in the logit life-table

---

16. See Brass, W. 'Mortality Estimation by Indirect Means', Expert Group Meeting on Mortality UNESOB Beirut, 1972. P_2/P_3 was used to locate the appropriate set of correction factors. This ratio was chosen for all villages because it is based on a larger number of ever-born live births than is the alternative ratio (P_1/P_2).
17. The 'African Standard' Model life table system is used here. It has been designed with the mortality patterns of Africa and Asia in mind. However the same analysis will be repeated using other model systems. For the 'African Standard' see Carrier, N. and Hobcraft, J. *Demographic Estimation for Developing Societies.* London Population Investigation Committee, 1971 pp. 70-85.
18. This range refers to the range of the boundary values of life-expectation in the model system. The actual range implied by the lx values themselves was of course smaller still.

system.[19] Then, assuming a one-parameter system, the averaged infant and childhood mortality figures were used to estimate rough values of life-expectation; these are given in Table 2.7. No claim is made that these estimates are exact. In particular they must be viewed against the range of mortality levels presented in Table 2.9. Similarly, they will have to be cross-checked against the mortality estimates resulting from questions on adult mortality. However, it must be said that the general order of these estimates are much as one would expect, given the corresponding estimates of life expectation for the relevant national populations.[20] Moreover the estimates have the advantage of referring to the specific units under study. As can be seen from Table 2.7 life expectation in Bogamuwa is estimated to be in the mid-sixties. The estimates for Viyalo and Taita are 48 and 52 years respectively. The estimate for Ramdaua is very low - 27 years. It is possible that this is marginally on the low side - adult mortality may be relatively lighter - but it is worth noting that stable population analysis on the relevant census district data also gives a very low estimate of life expectation for 1961.[21]

Finally, estimates of the village crude birth and death rates were made using the one-parameter model life tables corresponding to the estimated life expectancies; the 'estimates' of total fertility i.e. the mean parity values for women aged 40-49,[22] and lastly the age-sex distribution of the five largest villages.

The estimates of crude birth rates (CBR) were given in Table 2.5. The village with the highest CBR is Ramdaua. The two East African communities are estimated to have crude birth rates of around 50 per thousand. However, it should be noted that these estimates make no allowance for men and women absent from the villages, and we have seen that there are indications of such absence on the part of both males and females, particularly in

---

19. For this life-table system, see Brass, W. *et al*, *op.cit.* pp. 130-135. The resulting estimates of overall mortality (life expectation) refer to the recent past. Averaging the responses of all women (15-45) to the question on child-survivorship would probably not alter the estimates greatly (see Table 2.9) but the particular lx values used were thought to be slightly more reliable.

20. This is not true for the estimate for Ramdaua village, which is well below the All-India life expectation at birth.

21. The stable population analysis was actually applied prior to the initial period of fieldwork, and resulted in an estimate of 29.7 years. It was interesting to see these initial indications of very heavy mortality confirmed by the fieldwork questioning.

22. For the sake of convenience, the age-specific weighting of fertility used was the same for every village. It was the 'High-fertility Broad-peak' model distribution, given by the U.N. See United Nations, *Population Bulletin No. 7*. United Nations, New York, 1965, p. 110.

Viyalo. The lowest crude-birth rate is that of Bogamuwa; again, given the likelihood of some recent fertility decline in this village, the current value may well be lower.

Table 2.7 presents the estimates of the crude death rate. Not surprisingly this is estimated to be lowest in Bogamuwa (8.7) and highest in Ramdaua (37.1).

Lastly, Table 2.8 gives the associated estimates of the crude rate of natural increase (i.e. the crude birth rates minus the crude death rate). Taita and Viyalo are estimated to be growing very fast - at well over 3% per annum. Rampur is estimated to be increasing at 2.5% per annum, while Ramdaua is estimated to be growing at 1.9% per annum. Bogamuwa's estimated growth rate is only slightly below that of Ramdaua. However, as mentioned previously, it is likely that fertility is in fact currently lower in Bogamuwa than is assumed in making this estimate i.e. the population may well be growing at a slower rate than the estimated 1.9% per annum.

It is worth stressing that none of these further calculations has altered the conclusions arrived at through the analysis of the baseline data. The additional analysis has merely translated the data into estimates expressed in terms of conventional demographic variables (e.g. life expectation), and has only served to confirm our previous analysis and conclusions.

Summary and Discussion

In summary, this paper has made use of two sets of information to estimate and compare demographic parameters in the villages studied in this population project. It has shown that there is a considerable amount of variation among the villages with respect to these parameters.

The Sri Lankan village of Aluthgama-Bogamuwa is particularly interesting. To begin with, by all measures it has the lowest levels of fertility of any of the villages studied. Moreover fertility has been relatively low for some considerable period of time: women aged 40-49 have had on average 3.6 live births. Again, life expectation in Bogamuwa is estimated to be around 65 years i.e. the highest of any of the seven villages studied. Not surprisingly Bogamuwa has the lowest dependency burden, and the oldest age-structure.

In some respects the demography of Delumgoda is akin to that of Bogamuwa. Both fertility and mortality are relatively low - although they have not yet reached the levels prevailing in Bogamuwa. Moreover, unlike Bogamuwa, fertility levels in Delumgoda have declined from previously high levels: women aged 40-49 have had on average 6.5 live births per woman. Again the age-structure of Delumgoda's population is comparatively old - although not as old as that in Bogamuwa. The dependency ratios and rates of population growth in these two villages are comparatively low.

If the mean number of children surviving per woman is taken as a proxy for the rate of natural increase, then the Nigerian village of Umueke is growing at a slower rate than the two Kenyan villages. Fertility is high in Umueke, but not as high as in the Indian villages or in Taita and Viyalo. One is tempted to hypothesize that over the years out-migration has had a limiting effect on fertility levels. Certainly there is such migration out of Umueke, and this is one factor behind the village's very high dependency rate (96). The second factor controlling the natural growth of Umueke's population is a very high level of mortality: 27% of all live births to women aged 15-49 were reported as dead. The data suggest that only Ramdaua experiences a higher level of mortality.

The fastest growing of the seven village populations are Viyalo and Taita. Both the analysis in this paper, and the background census data, suggest that these two villages are growing at a rate in excess of 3% per annum. If these high rates continue then the populations will double approximately every twenty years. These rates of natural increase are particularly high, firstly because in both villages fertility is extremely high - the mean parity of women aged 40-49 is 7.9 in Taita and 8.6 in Viyalo - and secondly, because mortality levels in both villages are relatively low. Indeed as a group they are second only to those in Bogamuwa and Delumgoda - life expectation is estimated to be approximately 52 years in Taita and 48 years in Viyalo. One final result regarding these two villages is that in both the dependency ratio is very high. Viyalo in particular seems to have experienced heavy out-migration of both males and females in the economically active age range.

Finally, we can summarize the situation with regard to the Indian villages (Ramdaua and Rampur). To begin with, we can note that in neither are there any obvious signs of major out-migration. Although the dependency ratios are high, they are in fact lower than in Taita, Viyalo or Umueke. Again the mean parity values for women aged 40-49 are high in both villages - 7.0 in Rampur, and 7.7 in Ramdaua - but they are not quite as high as those in Taita and Viyalo. However, mortality in both Rampur and Ramdaua is much higher than the levels experienced in Taita and Viyalo. Life expectation is estimated at around 44 years in Rampur, and is certainly much lower in Ramdaua. It is primarily these high levels of mortality that limit the growth of population in Rampur, and to an even greater extent in Ramdaua.

In conclusion, although the estimates presented in this paper must be regarded tentatively, it is nevertheless clear that meaningful measures of fertility, mortality and population growth can be obtained in a situation typical of those in which anthropological field studies are conducted. The villages discussed in this paper vary widely with respect to these basic demographic parameters and it is apparent that such demographic information can be so important that no anthropological fieldwork can really afford to ignore it. Anthropological-demographic studies are made possible through the continual development of analytical techniques, and the advantages that accrue from the fieldworker's social immersion in the community under study. It is to be hoped that anthropologists will maintain an interest in 'measuring' fertility, mortality and migration, and that in addition they will continue to put flesh and blood on demographic statistics.

PART 2

CULTURE AND FERTILITY

CHAPTER 3

THE TRADITIONAL CULTURAL INVENTORY VERSUS THE ELITE ROADSIDE ECOLOGY

INTRODUCTION

It now seems generally accepted that there exists a relationship of mutual interdependence between economic and demographic changes. At the same time it must be realised that there is considerable economic differentiation both at international as well as intra-national level. The apparently commonsense inference that the poor should, as a matter of priority, reduce their birth rates if they wish to attain higher levels of living is a controversial matter. First of all, observed fertility behaviour has increasingly shown that the poorest tend to be least convinced by the 'logic' of this proposition. More significantly, there is even more divergence at the theoretical and policy levels. The 1974 Bucharest Population Conference tragically emphasised this rift. My paper is not meant to be a direct contribution to this debate; rather I seek to examine the issues from a different standpoint.

The debate so far has been based on theoretical macro concerns, whereas my argument here is based on empirical in-depth data collected at grass-root level. Rather than start with the question 'should or should not' the poor do this or that, the approach I pursue here is an examination of who does what and why. In other words the object is to identify who does or does not control fertility, under what conditions and why.

This research differs from most socio-demographic studies which analyse the problem in terms of indices such as income, education, occupation etc. Here emphasis is laid on one of the so far largely unexplored demographic determinants - culture in its entirety. By focusing on the micro-ecology I suggest it becomes apparent that there is a need for a balance within the total cultural dimension - i.e. between environment, technology and social organisation. A close look at the present day Maragoli society indicates that for most of its members this balance is lacking. It is this imbalance which helps to explain what otherwise is often regarded as irrational fertility behaviour. An analysis of these three dominant cultural variables forms the topic of this paper.

It is important to emphasise here that the attempt to introduce fertility control to the extent of significantly reducing macro growth rates would be a major intrusion into a vitally important area of a people's life - and a people who up until the end of the last century were living in a closed system. Central to this essay is the proposition that in such a closed system culture plays such a critical role that its analysis should take priority over any strictly demographic analysis. This is why I deal with this aspect first. I shall describe culture's functions in relation to its three major sub-divisions.

Culture has to grapple with the problems posed by the geophysical and social ecology if the collectivity has to survive. In order to perform this task it has to do at least two things. One, it has to evolve a technology (skills, knowledge and the ability to transmit these) which will enable the members to exploit and adapt their environmental resources. Two, to achieve this end, culture must harness the collectivity into some ordering - i.e. a social organisation. These three (environment, technology and social organisation) may in turn reshape the overall cultural system in the course of time. Here it is important to caution that there is not necessarily a one-way deterministic relationship between the environmental conditions and the operative cultural system.

Culture can then be seen as an inventory of solutions to the problems of the natural habitat, and here it is worth noting that the social ecology may pose even graver problems, e.g. hostile and belligerent neighbours may necessitate the development of a matching technology to cope with them. Similarly, technology has to wrestle with the most acute problem facing all members of the collectivity - mortality. Needless to say the efficiency of the cultural inventory in finding solutions to the problems of the ecology and the collectivity itself (power and economic struggles), depends on its ability to devise a fitting technology and an efficient social organisation. These theoretical considerations are of central importance to the rest of the essay, and I will now apply them to the Maragoli system.

Fertility in the Traditional Maragoli Culture

Here, as hinted above, culture is seen as an inventory of solutions to environmental and technological, as well as societal, problems. Though these variables are interlinked for the purpose of analysis I discuss each separately.

Environment

The Maragoli environment was relatively benign in terms of climate, altitude, rainfall, land fertility and man/land ratio. The social environment was somewhat less favourable; there were sworn ethnic enemies to the south (the Nyangori and Luo) and to the east (the Tiriki). The perennial source of hostilities was competition for the two major resources - fertile land and livestock.

Technology

The environment was amenable to an agrarian as well as a pastoral economy. In the event they were bi-cultural, with agriculture as the dominant feature (Wagner, 1956:39). They did not develop motor or animal power, consequently human labour was vital. Although the technological implements were very rudimentary they succeeded in extracting an agricultural surplus, e.g. they stored the harvest until the next crop to offset crop failure and famine was very rare (Wagner *op.cit:* 61-2). They appreciated the soil requirements of different crops and practised crop rotation. This is reflected in their social organisation by a scattered land-holding system. They also used fertilizers (e.g. compost) although cow dung was prohibited (Wagner *op.cit:* 26). Here it should be noted that all members falling within the same social category had equal access to technological knowledge and skills (e.g. male youth camps during circumcision). In this sense it was an egalitarian system.

Harnessing the environment is not the only concern of technology. More important still, given physical survival as the major objective of the collectivity, effective techniques were needed to wrestle with the gravest threat - death. The Maragoli appear to have had only rudimentary knowledge of how to combat their high mortality. In view of this they chose the only way to ensure their survival; they compensated for their high mortality by a complex network of fertility-inducing social mechanisms.

Social Organisation

The basic unit was the residential patrilineal corporate exogamous kin group, the clan. Here I concentrate only on those elements which have a specific demographic significance. It was egalitarian in the sense that it minimized privilege (the age-grade system ensures that in due time age as such confers certain benefits). Thus, the critical resource - land - was 'owned' by the clan; individuals and categories exercised 'rights' according to certain principles of allocation. There were two important ecological factors. As there were belligerent neighbours, social organisation had to cope with them. In the event, the Maragoli opted for an acephalous political structure in which the defence and conquest of land and livestock lay squarely on the clans. The clan was in turn divided into smaller kin groups of households.

The values inculcated were that each father tried to surround himself with as many youths as possible. He was unwilling to part with their energy, so to retain them he assured them of the two critical resources - land and cows. It was the duty of a father to give each of his sons a piece of land and the cows needed to marry a wife (Wagner, 1949:381). As land was still in plenty this was a relatively easy task. With regard to livestock the same egalitarian principle held:- give the cows to as many heirs as possible and when marrying also spread them to many clans - hence never marry simultaneously two sisters.

Here we see how the cultural system evolved strong fertility inducing incentives. The married man needed many children - on the one hand male energy was vital to defend, exploit or even loot the two vital resources. On the other hand marrying off one's daughter brought in cows - hence the need for early female marriage. Furthermore, in a system where durable goods were scarce, and in the absence of a monetary medium of exchange, lasting capital was not developed, the father had little to pass on to his children, and his stake in the future was guaranteed by procreation. In the face of high filial mortality the best insurance for 'parental immortality' was prolific procreation.[1] In this system, then, to highlight the high social values for fertility a whole stream of institutions and rituals were evolved to symbolize these values. A few examples will suffice.

Early conception was desired and to ensure it took place young couples indulged in frequent sex, and a woman's capacity for sexual enjoyment was believed to be vital. During this period the man's brothers were allowed to have sexual access to his wife. There were also fertility rites (Wagner, *ibid:* 413). Conversely the system had mechanisms of fertility control. One was child-spacing by prohibiting sex for a mother during lactation, and this period was extended. Infanticide was also practised in certain cases where the survival of the baby was regarded as a threat to the collectivity. For example, babies resulting from incest were killed; babies whose mothers died during parturition were also left to die. The sociological fact here is the context in which the life of a baby was legitimately terminated. However, this in itself does *not* provide a valid basis for arguing for or against the introduction of the fertility reductions under discussion here.

To recapitulate a few points raised so far. It has been argued that the Maragoli cultural system evolved a relatively efficient technology and social organization to exploit the environment. This technology was easily available to all the members but its failure to reduce mortality was countered by the high values attached to fertility and the social mechanisms inducing it. There was then a balance between the external environment, technology and the internal social organization. More importantly, all were culture specific in the sense that they were evolved in a closed system.

The whole process of 'modernization' can therefore be defined as the introduction of new cultural inventories of solutions to problems many of which arose out of changing conditions. This caused disequilibria in the ecological, technological and social organizational sub-systems. This essay is an attempt to show that in some ways the ecology has changed, thereby rendering obsolete some of the traditional technological and social organizational institutions. Who has benefited or been disadvantaged by the introduction of new technologies, and how? Is the present-day social organization selective in its choice of technology and how about its mechanisms of exploiting and allocating resources?

---

1. For a full analysis of this concept see Ssennyonga, J. in Epstein and Jackson, 1975.

Some General Observations

Environment and Technology in Maragoli (1975)

The major ecological changes occurred when, say, gold was discovered in the area in 1931 and the subsequent land alienation for this purpose. Again, the introduction of new vegetation and the harnessing of rivers to generate piped water are also important changes. On the social side the 'freezing' of ethnic hostilities and even more the introduction of resettlement schemes (by 1935, 4000 Maragoli were settled in Nyangori alone) must be taken into account. Institutions which were geared to a situation of constant warfare now became obsolete. For example, few fathers may need many sons around them to defend them today.

On the technological level, perhaps the most significant factor is education and its rewards. A western elitist system of education almost overnight brought wide differences in lifestyles, levels of living and, above all, world view. The Maragoli are ranked second in Kenya in terms of spending on education but as pointed out elsewhere, few are able to get it, let alone its benefits.[2] One other pertinent factor is the soaring educational inflation. A look at the salaries of the lucky few shows that they are not commensurate with the educational levels attained. Those who did eight years at school by 1960 for instance, because of the historical fact of the date of national independence, got jobs which even 'A level' graduates cannot get today. The 'O level' graduates are finding it very difficult to get jobs and are the most alienated category, and a growing menace because their education in no way equipped them for their rural environment. On the other hand, education has enabled them to glean other cultural inventories which are inaccessible to their rural uneducated mates.

Other technological novelties include agricultural implements such as tractors, new crop varieties, artificial fertilizers, techniques of planting, animal husbandry, and the use of extension services. Then there are the infrastructural services - telephone, electricity, post office, TV, radio, the press, clean water, etc. Perhaps more important is the use and availability of medical services. The introduction of a political superstructure during Kenya's colonial period aimed at a complete break with the traditional socio-political organization. However, certainly at grass-root levels, there is an important element of continuity persisting.[3]

Perhaps the most radical transformation was the introduction of new land laws. The clan no longer 'owns' the land, but it is

---

2. For a ranking in terms of education for all Kenya see ILO, 1972:pp.78-79, Employment, Incomes and Equality (Geneva).
3. Evidence of this is the office of the *Ligutu* in the sublocations.

all divided up under 'title' holders who 'own' it. There are no such safeguards as land ceiling and the legal land bottom is at best fictional.[4]

Maragoli culture used to stress co-operation, whereas the new economic opportunities emphasise competition. This new development resulted in a misfit within the social system: only the privileged few are now in a position to take advantage of the new technologies, while the majority have to rely on the traditional closed system's cultural inventories, at least in managing the major life crises - thanks to the resilience of the traditional system.

In one important respect, the new technology succeeded in controlling mortality-inducing factors, but not yet significantly enough to eradicate the people's fear of the threat to parental immortality - particularly infant and child mortality. On the other hand, the new technology does not appear to have been successful in its essential tasks of providing shelter and food for everybody. The traditional system precluded economic and social destitution, for example there were lands under the clan leader which were communally tilled to grow food for the aged and needy.

With reference to fertility, it is essential to stress here that the traditional system *had never had to cope with the strains generated by human numbers outstripping resources*. Such strains are a typically modern phenomenon. Therefore to look into the traditional cultural inventory for a solution would be an exercise in futility. Second, the proposed strategy of reducing fertility as a solution to food or resources shortages is also alien to such an inventory. Consequently, to ask a person who is operating with a traditional cultural inventory to adopt such a novel strategy is likely to be futile. These are generalised propositions; specific empirical data need to be examined in this context.

Here I describe the situation under the headings: economy, land and fertility. It will be shown that the introduction of new technologies as well as social organisational forms has not only exacerbated the economic differentials but has also brought with it a mechanism with an internal dynamism which systematically creates a downward spiral for some, while pushing others up the socio-economic ladder.

The Economy

The general characteristics have been described earlier. Only additional summary statistics are presented here. To understand the economic processes one has of necessity to go beyond the sub-location. The factors that explain and cause the sharp economic differentiation are largely external, especially the

4. For example 90% of the registered land-holdings in my research villages are below the official land-bottom of three acres.

TABLE 3.1

Economic stratification

Strata*	Households		Individuals		Average size of household
	Numbers	Percentage	Numbers	Percentage	Numbers
I	20	7.0	140	9.0	7.0
II	14	4.0	73	5.0	5.2
III	180	59.0	1018	65.0	5.7
IV	91	30.0	331	21.0	3.6
Total	305	100.0	1562	100.0	5.1

* The criteria for selecting these different strata were:

a) Type of residence
b) Available acreage
c) Assets
d) Wage and salaried income
e) Household composition

I did not construct a weighting index, but in the process of categorising households it became apparent that there is a coincidence between cash and other sources of income: the higher the cash earnings the greater the value of assets possessed as can be observed from the following tables.

TABLE 3.2

Regular cash income* p.a. by stratum

Strata	Households		Income in Kenya shillings p.a.	
	No. in sample	Percentage	Total	Average per household
I	14	70.0	259,120	18,508
II	13	92.6	122,710	9,439
III	64	35.6	146,534	2,289
IV	15	16.5	6,200	413
Total	106	34.8	534,564	Overall average 5,043

* The incomes refer to those cash earnings which could be reliably established. In practice, they refer to wages, salaries or other sources of regular cash incomes. In many instances they include wages earned in urban and industrial centres where the male household head may be working while the wife, children and other dependents live in the rural areas.

The figures do not reflect total incomes because subsistence produce, rents, etc. were not included. Consequently the table underestimates the earnings of particularly the top stratum who possess more valuable assets.

TABLE 3.3

Animal husbandry - distribution by stratum

Strata	Cows			Sheep			Goats		Pigs
	Numbers	Percentage	Average per household	Numbers	Percentage	Average per household	Numbers	Percentage	Numbers
I	72	17.0	3.6	14	35.9	.7	5	8.9	0
II	25	6.0	1.8	6	15.4	.4	1	1.8	0
III	258*	61.0	1.4	17	43.6	.1	43	76.8	4
IV	65+	16.0	0.7	2	5.1	.02	7	12.5	0
Total	420++	100.0	1.5	39	100.0	.12	56	100.0	4

* This figure excludes 25 cows which some members in this stratum 'caretake' for others.

\+ This figure excludes seven cows also under 'caretaker' arrangements. Most of these cows in fact belong to those in the upper strata.

++ The grand total therefore is 450 (two belong to people who are outside the sublocation and have been discounted).

TABLE 3.4

Poultry* by stratum

Strata	Chickens Nos.	Chickens %	Average No. per Household	Ducks Nos.	Ducks %	Turkeys Nos.	Quails Nos.
I	160	12.9	8	35	60	2	0
II	61	4.9	4.4	0	0	0	0
III	790	63.8	4.4	20	34.5	11	15
IV	227	18.3	2.5	3	-	0	5
Total	1238	100	4	58	100	13	20

* The data refer only to adult birds and ignore their sex.

ability to get a job in one of the major urban and industrial centres. It can safely be estimated that 90% of the Maragoli adult males have worked (usually as manual workers) outside the village, but this is always a temporary phenomenon as their place of eventual or forced retirement is the ethnic homeland. On the basis of cash income, property, land, education and family size, four strata have been isolated (see Table 3.1).

It is significant that the average regular cash income of a household in the top stratum is almost 45 times more than that of one in the lowest stratum. Assuming that the sample data on regular cash income are representative (i.e. for each stratum), if one aggregates the income per stratum as well as for all strata, one arrives at the following proportions. The top stratum, which represents 9% of the population, earns 38% of the total regular cash income, whereas the lowest stratum, accounting for 21% of the population gets only 3% of the gross total (see Tables 3.1 and 3.2). The existence of this wide gap between the richest and the poorest is consistently revealed in the distribution of other economic assets (see Tables 3.3 and 3.4).

TABLE 3.5

Differential access to land

Area	Registered land titles	Registered owners	Households	Mulimi* holders
Hectares	Nos.	Nos.	Nos.	Nos.
Less than 0.26	52	43	32	58
0.26 - 0.49	73	73	63	79
0.5 - 0.9	93	92	106	123
1.00 - 1.4	42	43	45	59
1.5 - 1.9	20	20	31	40
2.00 - 2.4	4	4	3	5
2.5 - 2.9	2	2	5	5
3.00 - 3.4	4	3	5	8
Totals	290	280	290	377

* Mulimi holders have rights in land by virtue of their specific relationship with the registered owners; they are the actual cultivators.

Land

Land data (Table 3.5) were not analysed in terms of the four economic strata, because in many cases the sons of one single man, all having land rights on the same land holding, may be in four different strata depending on their education and jobs.

The top stratum on average hold land as single households on a single title basis and have several land holdings, some as far apart as 60-70 miles. The fact that land prices are soaring means that only the rich can afford to buy more land and the poor are tempted to sell. In Viyalo sub-location the current price of half an acre is usually 3,000 Kenyan shillings (about £200 sterling), and this is eight times more than the estimated annual regular cash income of those in the poorest stratum.

Furthermore, the services of the experimental Special Rural Development Programme, which include treated water, telephones and electricity, are all roadside facilities which are very difficult to exploit for anyone residing far away from the road. The better off are responding to this new pull factor by buying land near or along the main road. They are the only telephone and private post office box renters, as well as the prospective subscribers to the projected electricity extension (some have already wired their houses in anticipation). I have described this phenomenon as the elite roadside ecology.

Initially I attempted to correlate fertility characteristics with the economic strata but I soon came up against problems of immense proportions. A few examples may suffice here. First, there are only small numbers in the top two strata and this creates demographic analytical impasses (e.g. an uneven age spread). Second, many of those in the top economic stratum improved their economic standards either towards or at the end of their fertility. Third, polygamy complicates the issues in several ways. Some men married women who were previously married to men of lower economic strata. In one case a single man has three wives but their household differentials have nothing to do with their fertility. It is a matter of favouritism.

Land is perhaps the variable that is least amenable to this sort of exercise. A father may have one hectare of land registered under his name, but he may subdivide it among his three or four sons who may be in three or four different economic strata. There was also a methodological limitation, namely the fact that the data were collected on a *de facto* residential population. In a high out-migration area such as Maragoli, this generates further constraints. On the one hand it hides the dependence factor, for example pupils at boarding schools outside the sub-location. On the other hand it involves problems of estimating the cash earnings of households or other near kin urban workers - most rural women do not know their husbands' wages. Furthermore, some urban migrants have dependants they

TABLE 3.6

Regular and casual employment* by stratum

Strata	Total no. of households	Regular Employment: No. of households	Regular Employment: Percentage	Casual Wage Labour: No. of households	Casual Wage Labour: Percentage
I	20	20	100	1	5
II	14	13	93	0	0
III	180	105	58	55	31
IV	91	11	12	28	31
Total	305+	149	48.8 (overall average)	84	27.5 (overall average)

* As can be seen from Table 3.7, the employment opportunities are very bleak within the sub-location, hence the high proportion of male out-migration.

\+ Since most of these incomes are earned away from home, a considerable amount is consumed at the places of work, thereby reducing the cash flow into these rural homes.

TABLE 3.7

Household member in casual wage labour by sex and stratum

Sex	Stratum I	Stratum II	Stratum III	Stratum IV	Total	Percentage
M	0	0	9	15	24	32.4
F	0	0	34	16	50	67.6*
Total	0	0	43	31	74	100

* The high proportion of women in this labour force is a function of the high male out-migration rate as well as the land tenure system.

may be unwilling to reveal, such as 'temporary' wives. Lastly, since only five or so couples ever took any voluntary (i.e. excluding sterilization for health reasons) fertility controls, the utility of such a laborious exercise became more questionable.

Instead, I divided the universe into three basic categories.

a) The traditional ecological stratum; i.e. those who have not attempted fertility control and are unlikely to do so without radical changes in their socio-economic environment.

b) The elite roadside ecological stratum. These are drawn from the top economic stratum although there are indications that some couples from the upper middle economic stratum (particularly the younger ones) will also at least use terminal fertility controls.

c) The 'ever present' young migrant elite - the sons and daughters of the present rural elite. These are the first to make full use of contraceptives as pre-marital and marital fertility controls. However the majority of these are away either in urban or educational centres. Since they are all Maragoli, they are the ever present migrants. Now a brief description of each category.

The Traditional Ecological Stratum

This consists of predominantly agrarian subsistence peasants with no regular earnings. Those who go elsewhere in search of jobs are mostly male, unskilled wage labourers (see Table 3.6). Their household agricultural produce can meet their food needs for only eight or even less months in any one year. Since their urban earnings are so meagre, they suffer an annual slow and quiet famine between February and May.[5] As their landholdings are usually so tiny the fathers are finding it increasingly difficult to subdivide the land, so they delay the painful exercize. Meanwhile they dig, harvest and cook together, i.e.

---

5. In this context the following account is relevant: I settled down in the village on August 28 but by mid September I had already learned of the hard days of the *enzala* or famine, which occurs between February and May. The food grains harvested in December have run out and the next harvest begins in May. It is certainly a tragedy that officialdom (e.g. agricultural reports etc.) say nothing about this annual plight. But this is a fact which everyone in the village knows. Perhaps the most striking illustration of the people's grave concern was a young schoolgirl's graphic expression. Every year just before Christmas the women and girls paint the walls of the houses and write Christmas and other general good wishes on the outer walls. The message on one of the walls in a poor home read, "You are welcome but no food". I cannot forget how on two different occasions as I arrived to carry out interviews the women informed me that they had not eaten anything for three days.

TABLE 3.8

Education expenses per student p.a.

Items	Primary Schooling (1-4 years)* K.Sh.	Secondary[+] schooling K.Sh.
Building Fund (Fees)	77	920
Activities Fund	3	-
School Watchman	5	-
Lunch	-	200
Transport	-	260
Clothes[++]	65	205
Total	150	1,585

* The first four years of primary schooling are free, but charges occur.

[+] The figures refer to an *Harambee* (self-help) school.

[++] These totals refer to girl students and are slightly less for boys.

the parental and their filial marital units. As already mentioned there is no clear fit between the four socio-economic strata and the three ecological categories; however, there are signs of a coincidence between the traditional ecological stratum and the two lowest socio-economic strata.

Compared with the other categories they experience a higher infant and child mortality rate and end up with less surviving children, consequently their parental immortality concerns are very great. In one extreme case a woman bore 23 children and only three had survived by the time she was 60 years old. Cultural practices and beliefs regulating fertility are still very strong for this category. Here I can only cite a few examples.

Several times I came across cases where women had long spells of infertility. Very often they would explain this by saying that an aunt or some other relative had pronounced a curse. In other cases some would say they were experiencing frequent bleeding - *okutaaza*. In one case a woman told me that she started bleeding after a month's pregnancy and this went on for four years when she eventually gave birth to the baby. It is important to note here that the solutions to problems of infertility are usually those provided by the traditional cultural inventory. For example, one who believes she was cursed by her aunt will arrange for a reconciliation and the curse is then lifted. On the other hand, fertility is a gift from God, who alone can decide how many children one may have. Hence it is not up to man to decide, much less control, the number of children. In this respect God is part and parcel of their ecological system; his role is of cardinal importance.

The residence pattern puts the young mother and her baby under the direct control of the man's mother, who usually acts as midwife. This mother will be the first to complain if the wife does not conceive quickly. The sanctions for female infertility effectively reduce her to a social and economic status of a minor. For example a man is entitled to divorce an infertile woman and demand the return of the bride wealth, especially the cows. Again, a woman's legal (traditional) rights and access to land are strictly marital.

This category, which includes the majority of Maragoli, encounters great difficulties in taking advantage of the first four years of education which are legally free. In fact costs are involved (see Table 3.8), which make it virtually impossible for the poorest to send their children to school.

This socio-economic setting thus reveals an ecology in which the members have very scarce resources with a skewed distribution. It is important to re-emphasize here the fact that these people have been given little access to modern technology. This makes it difficult for them to plan their resources effectively because they are not even sure of meeting tomorrow's needs. They then tend to discount the future in terms of worldly as opposed to other-worldly rewards. This distinction is necessary because the Maragoli are a very religious people and attach

TABLE 3.9

Mortgages involving land estates

Size of land (Hectares)	Loan (in K.Shs.)	Interest (p.a.)	Date	Lender
1.4	5,200	Not stated	June 1974	Agricultural Finance Corporation
0.39	4,000	Not stated	March 1974	Kenya Commercial Bank (Kakamega)
.41	10,000	9½%	Sept. 1973	Barclays International Limited (Nairobi)
.8	30,000	Not stated	Aug. 1973	Not stated
.7	40,000	10%	March 1974	Kenya Commercial Bank (Kakamega)
1.9	30,000	9½%	Feb. 1974	Barclays International Limited (Nairobi)
.27	3,000	6½%	Jan. 1974	Kakamega Trade Development Joint Board
.08	4,000	Not stated	Nov. 1974	Standard Bank Limited (Nairobi)
3.4	10,000	Not stated	Sept. 1974	Standard Bank Limited (Nairobi)

great importance to 'life after death'. Here the time series are important when discussing their deferred gratification and opportunity-cost considerations.

Obviously these characterizations are not equally true for all the individuals in this category as a certain degree of socio-economic differentiation can be seen from the tables showing the distribution of incomes and other economic assets. The crucial fact is that they have a very limited capacity to change their ecology. This is the central bastion of my inference that, not surprisingly, they have not attempted to solve the typically modern problem of numbers outstripping resources by an alien cultural inventory solution - that of fertility control. Let us now have a look at those who *have* adopted this solution.

The Elite Roadside Ecology Stratum

Genealogically they are the sons of the first generation to have had access to some elementary modern technology (especially education and skills) which enabled them to secure paid jobs. A few eked out some savings and educated one or two sons, or even bought land. These sons were thus equipped with relatively higher technological benefits which in turn opened up new and higher avenues for them. One of the distinctive manifestations of their acquisition of more powerful status is their movement away from their paternal compound to establish new homes along or near the road. This sums up their social economic and fertility behaviour differentials.

The new residential pattern marks a changed relationship with their immediate clan kinsmen. They have more land and hence need more labour which their less fortunate kinsmen would willingly offer, but as this would mean the perpetuation of the traditional sibling and filial ideology of equality in property allocation, they find it more convenient to recruit labour on a contractual basis with a patron/client element. It is significant, therefore, that none of the housewives in the top and upper middle economic strata are engaged in casual labour. They also have monopolistic access to the modern institutions of capital formation; e.g. they are the only persons who can risk mortgaging off some of their scattered land holdings to obtain loans (see Table 3.9).

Their fertility behaviour also shows a departure from the traditional ecology. They are the first to use fertility controls, albeit terminally, i.e. after getting a high fertility - on average 9-10 children. Their close connections with the mortality-reducing institutions (e.g. two nurses and a doctor are 'children' of this elite), coupled with their superior technology, arms them more efficiently to deal with and minimise the fears of 'total parental death'.

Though this elite stratum differs somewhat from any of the socio-economic strata discussed already, it does display many of the characteristics of the upper two strata. Briefly, this stratum represents the success story of a modern ecological process; they reshape their environment by manipulating the new technologies and the new social organizational framework. They are therefore in a position to bequeath a more lasting legacy to their children who are going to benefit even better from it.

The Ever-present Young Migrant Elite

My data on this category are as yet incomplete, but they can illustrate a basic trend. For the present I will limit myself to a few examples of a generalised nature.

These young elite migrants have attained a relatively high level of education, on average, of at least 14 or more years for both sexes. This gives them immense advantages, especially in terms of access to alternative cultural inventories. But in fertility behaviour it is important to point out a significant sex differential. Of the 20 females (15-24 age group) in this category, only two are married (10%, compared to 31.7% for the total universe age group figure). On the other hand, of the 13 males in this age group (for whom I have reliable information) nine have caused premarital pregnancies, only one of which resulted in marriage. The girls are usually from lower economic strata and are forced to discontinue their education. These pregnancies often occur during school holidays. Here it is pertinent to note that the Family Planning programmes concentrate their services only on married persons.

These elite sons and daughters are an invaluable asset to their parents. For many rural parents, education is perhaps the most viable single investment, as well as being a form of old-age insurance. In one family, for example, the five employed sons and daughters have worked out an arrangement whereby they meet all the educational expenses of their younger three siblings, which involves a considerable expenditure, particularly on secondary schooling (see Table 3.8).

In return, the parental generation encourages, negotiates on behalf of, or even buys land for, their sons - usually along the road, for it is expected that these young professionals will eventually retire in their homeland. From this point of view their break with the traditional culture is not complete but they do exert considerable influence on the direction of the ecology. Perhaps one area where I expect conflict is the inheritance norms. The traditional rule is that the youngest male sibling inherits the father's house, and in the past he was also entitled to one of the polygamous wives (other than his mother). This fits well with the traditional ecology of rudimentary technology (e.g. thatched house and virtually no durable household property). But in an ecology where the household's residence may be its most valuable single asset (where it is permanent - bricks and corrugated roof as most houses in the top stratum are) this may cause tensions among male siblings. I suspect that this will lead to a change in inheritance rules. Alternatively, where the father can accumulate other economic assets he may easily spread them - a solution which those in the poorer strata cannot emulate. Perhaps this illustrates why I preferred to discuss the issues in terms of who does or does not do what and for what reasons.

Conclusion

The theme of this chapter can be summed up in the following propositions:

Firstly, the present day social system is the result of an uneasy mixture of the traditional and modern ecological processes. I have tried to show that for the vast majority in my universe, their role in the latter is peripheral in terms of influence and benefits.

Secondly, the modern adaptation to the changed socio-technological environment appears to be tragically inefficient if judged by the performance of its central tasks of producing and distributing food to all the members of the collectivity. Moreover, it fails to ensure maximum survival in terms of life expectancy and the transmission of a fitting and easily accessible technology, as well as a social organizational framework that safeguards the essential values of co-operation and equal opportunities for all. The worsening man-land ratio and the acute food shortages in a situation of unlimited competition serve as sad evidence of this. One further consideration agronomists may seriously examine is the animal growth rate in a situation of acute land shortage.

Thirdly, from a more strictly demographic point of view, we come to another characteristic, namely that there is *no* evidence to show that the current high crude birth rate is going to fall in the immediate future. The basis for this proposition rests on the fact that only a tiny proportion of the population are at all concerned with fertility controls, and even then only of a terminal nature. Moreover, there is a growing rate of premarital babies.

Fourthly, I have argued that it is not merely a statistical coincidence that those who use terminal methods of contraception are the ones who have been the greatest beneficiaries from the new ecological process. Their ability to change both their geophysical and social environment through a superior technology, thanks to the new social organization, goes hand in hand with their overall behaviour of which fertility is one aspect. Those who have the effective power to plan and control this process better are the ones who can also be expected to control their fertility. The available empirical data lead me to conclude that this has also been the observed case. The users are part and parcel as well as a by-product of this new ecological process. By contrast, those in the traditional ecological stratum are ill-equipped to resolve the resultant imbalance in the system. It may be due to the characteristic weakness of certain macro-statistical arrangements, and hence their 'logic', that those who are largely using solutions from a traditional cultural inventory are asked to have the same fertility behaviour as those who have adopted newer and more appropriate ecologies.

Finally, the theoretical and policy implications of these considerations are of immense proportions. The new ecological system appears to have an internal dynamism which of its very nature is bound to generate a downward spiral for the majority and an upward one for a tiny minority. If the desired goal is a more rational and equitable interdependence between demographic and socio-economic trends then more far-reaching strategies than the present 'patch-up' arrangements are required. To establish this viable interdependence we need to go beyond the conventional approach of analysing population trends in terms of specific selected indices such as education, income, urbanization and the like. This is why I suggest a 'system' approach which examines the interrelationship of all the variables forming the entire cultural dimensions of a society.[6]

---

6. During my fieldwork period a film was made in the village which followed this approach. The film, directed by Sandra Nichols, is named after the village - *Maragoli*.

CHART 3.1

VIYALO SUB-LOCATION 1974: AGE/SEX PYRAMID

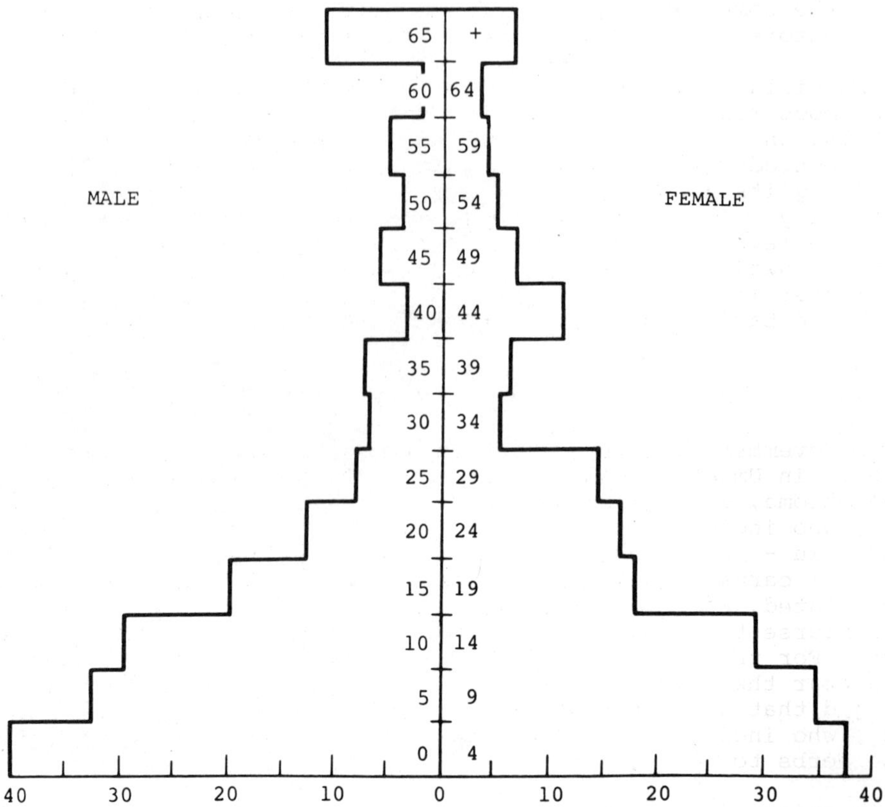

CHAPTER 4

CONTINUITY AND CHANGE: ABORTION AND FAMILY SIZE IN A NIGERIAN VILLAGE

INTRODUCTION

Umueke[1] is one of the eleven villages constituting the Agbaja Clan[2] - a territorial unit located in the Mbano Division of the East Central State, Nigeria. The Clan is also a kin unit since the component villages claim common descent from a pair of ancestors - a man called Ngalaba and his wife named Okpu-ite.

The villages function within the clan's umbrella set-up as autonomous maximal lineages, true to the much talked about egalitarian ethos of most Igbo. Thus the Clan is a somewhat loose confederation functioning as an ideological unit and affording its constituent villages some measure of social solidarity. The villages themselves are socially organised on two main levels - the extended family and the compound. The former constitutes a major lineage made up of several compounds. The latter is a minimal lineage and consists of many households which are basic independent economic units.

John and Ahudie: A Case of Abortion

In November 1974 the Ikpeamas, who constitute a minimal lineage in Umueke, lodged a complaint to the police against John Obioma, who was my chief research assistant. The complainants, who incidentally belong to the same major lineage - Umu-Dumuamaku - as the accused, alleged that on two occasions he had unlawful carnal knowledge of their daughter Ahudie. The girl, they stated, was under age and was lured into having sexual intercourse the first time by being invited home for dinner by John. For the second alleged sexual assault the girl was waylaid near the village stream - Nkwei. The Ikpeamas further alleged that after these affairs Ahudie became pregnant, and John, who incidentally is a herbalist, was obliged to administer some herbs to her with a view to effecting an abortion.

Abortion, it must be noted, was then a crime in Nigeria. Following the complaint, the police searched John's hut, removed some herbs for forensic analysis, and took him into custody.

---

1. The village was first studied between 1934-37 by Dr. M.M. Green who subsequently published her findings in *Igbo Village Affairs* (1964).
2. The other constituent villages are, Umu-Ofa, Abosi, Mgbam, Umu-Obia, Umu-Meke, Umu-Echele, Dinka, Umu-Chakwa, Umu-Imo and Umu-Duruaro.

Subsequently he was charged in court for seeking to procure an abortion. But what an irony: barely a year after John's arrest (December 1975) Nigeria's Federal Commissioner for Health mooted the legalisation of abortions.

John's trial lasted a period of six months, the last day of which saw a brief but lively debate between Defense and Prosecuting Counsel. John's Counsel began his somewhat marathon closing address by arguing that the swearing of 'sasswood oaths' at regular intervals is a salient feature of Umueke's socialization process. One of the oaths, he noted, forbids homicide, including abortion, and another prohibits incestuous sexual intercourse. Counsel further referred to the strong hold which superstition has over Umueke's society, and contended that his client, like most of his compatriots, would shudder at the thought of breaking the dreadful oaths. Touching on the various technical points raised by the prosecution, Defense Counsel submitted that sufficient evidence had not been adduced to sustain the charge against his client. He finally urged the court to acquit and discharge John. Shortly afterwards John's Counsel commented that it was about time that abortions were legalised. He noted that crude and clandestine abortions have brought enormous misery to millions of Nigerian women like Ahudie. He then called for a fuller application of scientific discoveries to improve the quality of life for the individual both at the national and family levels. Counsel finally contended that legalising abortion would be a bold and genuine attempt "to adapt to our modern environment with its somewhat unfamiliar demands".

In his reply, Prosecuting Counsel submitted that such modernising influences as Christianity and western education have for a long time vitiated the superstition prevalent in Umueke. Therefore belief in the supposed efficacy of 'sasswood oaths' may not be as strong in today's Umueke as Defense Counsel thought. He further argued that the village is hardly a Utopia, and so some of its members are bound to be deviants who would break societal norms - oaths or no oaths.

Speaking of abortion, Prosecuting Counsel conceded that the application of medical and other scientific knowledge should be maximized. He noted, however, that about 80% of Nigerians live in rural areas and that they hardly experience the 'modern environment' to which Defense Counsel alluded. He then declared: "If my learned friend thinks that free-for-all abortion is the latest scientific spin-off that could most effectively palliate the misery of a majority of Nigerian women, then he has got his recipe for the nation's socio-economic advancement very well warped." And that ended his submission.

In his ruling, the Magistrate reviewed the arguments advanced and the evidence adduced by both parties. He noted that the forensic analysis tendered by the Prosecution was inconclusive, and decided to resolve the resultant ambiguity in favour of the accused. John was thus acquitted and discharged. Turning to the debate on abortion, the Magistrate commended the candour with which it had been conducted, and informed both counsel rather humorously: "Neither of you has won or lost the debate."

John's arrest, and the chain of events which it triggered off, was easily the most eventful occurrence in the 13 months or so during which I lived in Umueke. Prior to my contact with John, the villagers were very suspicious of my intentions. As a result, whenever I put questions they either hedged or fobbed me off with unfulfilled promises to answer at a later time; occasionally they told downright lies. John's collaboration with me not only helped to overcome the respondent's resistance, but also enabled me to gain access to data which I would otherwise never have been able to gather. The improved relations with the villagers, which derived largely from John's social standing, continued until his arrest.

Thereafter, the villagers' resentment at the 'intrusion' of the police in their 'internal affairs' necessitated a repudiation of all things 'foreign' and 'external' - including my studies. In the prevailing circumstances, I had to suspend my systematic enquiries. However, the ensuing lull turned out to be a blessing in disguise. It afforded me the opportunity to observe more effectively the in-fighting and re-alignment prompted by the supervening crisis. This aftermath was indeed very revealing in terms of the dynamics of the social system.

John's arrest and trial present a classic 'social drama'. I use the episode as an illustration not only of the villagers cultural values, but also of the interplay between demography and other socio-economic change processes. By analysing the respective roles of the dramatis personnae involved in this case, I attempt to delineate spheres of persistence and change in the social system. I also attempt to lay bare some contradictions between the normative and the pragmatic rules that operate in the system.

The Colonial Past

Some twenty-six years after her initial research in Umueke, Dr. Green returned to the village. She observed (1964:ix) that some material changes had occurred in the urban areas of Igboland, whereas not much evidence of such changes existed in Umueke and other rural areas. One readily recalls Marechal Dumaurex, who in a reference to the courtiers of Louis XVII of France, remarked: "They have forgotten nothing and learned nothing".

Anthropological accounts abound which suggest that most pre-colonial African cities, like their counterparts elsewhere, developed materially at the expense of their outlying districts. Nevertheless, it seems that the very developmental imbalance discerned by Dr. Green is something of a systemic as well as institutional failure which derives from a colonial past. Forays of the British Army, which ushered in colonial rule in most of Igboland at the very beginning of this century, did not spread to

Umueke until about 1911. The advent of colonial rule prompted many structural changes, one of which was monetization of the village's economical system. The intrusion of cash influence precipitated a dual economy - the co-existence of subsistence and cash orientation. The latter was developed to feed primary agricultural products, like palm oil and kernel, to trading posts established by Europeans. From the depots the raw materials were exported to metropolitan centres in Europe. Most of the European merchants as well as the colonial administrators lived at the trading posts. Hence the stations were given priority in all allocation of development projects. Most of the erstwhile trading posts have evolved into current urban centres. The uneven development pattern laid down by the Europeans, which could very well be referred to as a 'false start', has persisted till now (c.f p.137). Hence, the relative backwardness of such rural areas as Umueke can largely be attributed to the urban bias of Nigeria's past and present development programmes.

It seems that Dr. Green's observation that there had not been much material change in Umueke is more obvious at societal rather than individual level. At the time of her return visit, the village, like most rural and urban areas in Nigeria, had had more than sixty years of colonial experience. This entailed, as indicated above, a link between the village economy and the national economic system, which in turn became absorbed within the world economy. The experience also brought about the advent, in 1924, of such new resources as western education, which later provided an alternative to agriculture as a means of achieving upward social mobility. I suggest that the sustained enthusiastic response of the Igbo to the innovations of the so-called colonial experience as discerned by Ottenberg (1959:130), brought them considerable material benefits. These were bestowed differentially, as will be illustrated later, in terms of the highly individualised competitiveness of the people observed by Levine (1966).

A perusal of Dr. Green's book readily indicates her somewhat group-oriented methodology, as well as her functionalist theoretical perspective. Her methodology tends to gloss over structural differentiations while her theoretical perspective tends to stress consensus and equilibrium, which in turn often under-rate the potential of the internal dynamics of a social system as change-stimulating factors.

By way of contrast to Dr. Green's approach, my study focuses more on the individual than the group - his/her interaction with other individuals in the society. I have taken the stance that the individual strives to take expressive actions, whilst working and playing with another, with a view to achieving the gratification which sharing the common identity of a corporate group brings. However, other interactions with other individuals often entail a conflict of interest. This is particularly so in the context of growing needs and dwindling resources. A rapidly growing population intensifies this conflict.

Umueke's *Weltanschauung*

Conversations between Umueke villagers, especially in moments of frustrated ambitions, are often replete with such millenary phrases as: "When I next venture into this world ...". This represents the people's belief in the phenomenon of re-incarnation. They manifest their world-view more overtly when births occur. One of the society's natal rites obliges the parents of the newly-born to enquire from a diviner about who has supposedly come back to life in the person of the baby. When the identity of the 'protégé' baby is thus established, the parents proceed to name the child appropriately after its spiritual 'progenitor'. The birth rite is a measure of cultural resilience, and not only prescribes but also regulates roles in the village's social system.

John, the accused in the abortion case, is thought to be a protégé of Dumamaku - the founding ancestor of the Umu-Dumamaku major lineage. John's prestigious social identity has been further enhanced by the fact that his is the head compound of the kin unit. He enjoys a somewhat jocular relationship with members of his lineage, and though still a young man himself he maintains a paternal image. Hence his Counsel felt free to submit at the trial that it would be utterly absurd to imagine that John would have sexual intercourse with Ahudie, who is his classificatory daughter.

John's social status, like most social positions, has rights, privileges, duties and obligations attached to it. But for the fact that he is still single at 27, John would have been the keeper of the Lineage 'Ofo' - the wooden staff of ritual authority. He would also have been enjoying the privilege of breaking Kola nuts at lineage meetings - a sign of ritual leadership.

John's marital status is not a unique case; there are several other young men of his age who are still unmarried. In 1956 the then Eastern Nigerian Government felt so concerned about escalating bridewealth that it initiated concerted legislative efforts to peg it down. In spite of these efforts, suitors today in Umueke and the surrounding area have to pay as much as £50 for an illiterate bride; £70 for a lady who has completed her primary education or learnt a trade like sewing or weaving; and £125 for one who has had a secondary education. The bridewealth is rather disproportionate considering that the average annual cash income per capita in Umueke is only about £22. The upward trend in bridewealth seems to be a reflection of the spiralling inflation that has gripped Nigeria's economic system. As a result of the escalating bridewealth many eligible bachelors like John are forced to postpone their marriage.

While the lineage waits for John to marry and thereby 'come of age', his uncle, Peter Elemai, has been appointed to bear the *Ofo*. This is to ensure the continued performance of the functional integrative purpose of the instrument. Peter thus takes John's place amongst other *Ofo* bearers designated *'Ama Ala'* - elders. Umueke, like most Igbo coroporate groups, is acephalous, its polity being diffused.[3] The village elders constitute a college that largely performs goal attainment functions by providing the rudiments of traditional government. Thus, government in Umueke is essentially gerontocratic.

In the past, age-grades featured prominently in the social system, and provided the framework for 'graduating' to the status of an elder. Today, the place of the age-grade is being taken by a new type of social organisation called the 'Youth'[4] which seems, from its structure and functions, to have been diffused from urban centres.

It must be emphasised that formulating the society's goals in traditional terms is not the exclusive privilege of the elders. Economic opportunities are open to all, and efforts like those of the successful farmer or trader are recognised and rewarded. Such elite entrepreneurs who are free-born are often admitted to the society's leadership irrespective of their age. But as stated before, the social system places a high normative premium on egalitarian values. Consequently, the honour of being invited to participate in village government is strictly achieved. That is to say, it dies with the person on whom it is conferred. His off-spring have to work hard to merit it in their own right. This egalitarian ethos conflicts, however, with Umueke belief in re-incarnation. As has been indicated with relation to John, his social prestige is largely the result of his being regarded as the re-incarnation of a prestigious ancestor.

Although there are thus some limitations to the egalitarian ethos among Umueke villagers, their traditional government in the society is not invested in one but in a coterie of wise and distinguished citizens.

Umueke's Census Data

At the time of the baseline studies in 1937, Umueke had an entire population of about 361, consisting of 360 residents and one 'permanent' out-migrant. But at the time of my enquiry in 1974/5 the village had increased to 543, made up of 357 residents and 186 non-residents (or out-migrants). It follows, therefore,

---

3. In this context, it should be noted that the small proportion of Igbo who claim to originate from the ancient Kingdom of Benin have a structured and centralised polity (see: Onwuazor, S.N. 1975:70).
4. There are about six youth organisations in the village, viz: Ahana, Chigozie, Egbe-Bere, Njoku, Idinanma and Sabastine. For a fuller account of the youth organisations see: Onwuazor, S.N. (1975): "The Declining Age-Grade System of Umueke" (an unpublished paper.

Table 4.1

Desired number of children and their sex composition

Household No.	Ideal Size	No. of boys	No. of girls
35a	12	8	4
18	8	5	3
23	8	6	2
76	8	4	4
30a	12	8	4
20	7	5	2
9	12	8	4
22	8	6	2
17	6	4	2
15	5	4	1
33	12	7	5
96	8	4	4
90	8	5	3
12	9	7	2
16a	15	10	5
5	7	5	2
78	12	8	4

Average size = 9.23 children
Preference for more boys 88%
" " " girls -
" " equal number of boys and girls 12%

that:

(a) the entire population had increased by 40-50%

(b) the resident population had declined, suffering a negative growth of about 1%

(c) the non-resident members had increased from 0.25% of the entire population to about 34%.

It is discerned that the population had been growing at an annual rate of 1% *on the average* since the baseline enquiry. It is also calculated that the society's Total Fertility Ratio (TFR) was 6.75 live births per woman. This readily suggests that the seemingly low growth rate was not necessarily applicable at the time of the re-study. In fact, the TFR indicates a much higher rate of growth.

A number of interrelated variables influence Umueke's population growth. Not even the considerable proportion of women within the ages 20-29 who live in towns or the spiralling bridewealth seems to have had much attenuating effect on Umueke's fertility trend. The following factors contribute to Umueke's high fertility.

1. High fertility ideology. The people of Umueke (and most Igbo) give their children the name *"Nwakaego"*, which means "A child is more precious than money". They also call their children *"Igwebuike"*, literally meaning "The crowd is strength". Similarly they have an adage which goes: *"Onwe mmadu ka onwe ego"*, which when given a literal interpretation reads "He that has people is greater than one who has money". The two names, as well as the adage, manifest the people's joy at, and conceptualise their rationale for, a large family. Table 4.1 indicates that the heads of households in my stratified random sample desire *on the average* about 9.23 children. As one of the motivations for achieving this comparatively large number, a housewife is honoured and rewarded by her husband after her tenth live birth. On such an occasion a goat or even a cow is slaughtered to give a feast. On the other hand, if the wife is deemed to be not 'pulling her weight', her husband could exert some sanctions. For example, if the wife fails to bear a male child, her husband could 'keep on trying' with her while constantly reminding her that she has not 'gained a foothold in the lineage'. If, on the other hand, the problem is that the woman is altogether barren, her husband could choose to marry another wife. Both options tend to increase fertility. This emphasis on high fertility helps to explain the normative condemnation of abortion, as exemplified in the court case discussed earlier.

2. Support from children. A large number of children is sought for a variety of reasons. First, most parents are not aware that the village's mortality is reducing, so they still consider it safer to have many children in order to ensure that at least some will survive. Second, children represent a means

of social security. This derives from the expectation that it behoves children to take care of their elderly parents. Thus the larger the number of children, the greater the 'duty of care' and the security accruing from it.

Third, children could make a significant difference in terms of labour force and income, despite the low conceptual stress on their productivity.

3. The importance of male offspring. Although children of both sexes are counted as a blessing from God and are welcome, male children are 'more welcome' than females, as can be gleaned from Table 4.1. True, children of both sexes accord their parents 'immortality'. But in Umueke's patrilineal society, only males can perpetuate the lineage. In this context, male children are light-heartedly referred to as 'home'. On the other hand, although females bring in a considerable income in terms of bridewealth, they are referred to as 'away'. This manifests the feeling of deprivation the family nurses when a daughter gets married and has to leave her natal home, since marriage is viri-local.

The great importance attached to having male offspring puts additional pressure on couples who have only daughters to continue producing children until they manage to get one or two sons.

4. The gambling factor. As a response to poverty both at societal and individual levels, the villagers tend to produce many children in the hope that one of them at least will eventually be successful.

5. Ethnicity. Nigeria is a culturally heterogeneous nation, constituted by a myriad of distinct corporate groups categorised linguistically under three major tribes - the Igbo, Hausa and Yoruba. These tribes have been locked in ethnic rivalry since the mid-forties or thereabout, motivated largely by a desire to control the nation's central government. Constitutionally, the much contested political authority derives from numerical strength - the majority rule. It is no wonder, therefore, that an accurate census has been the most battered casualty of the ethnic feud. Since independence in 1960, Nigeria has had to count its population three times and each time has been unable to produce reliable statistics. On each occasion it was discovered that various groups had bloated their numbers as part of their retribalisation strategy for gaining control of the central government.

Conceivably, one would be tempted to think that the people of Umueke are insulated from the census politics by virtue of their low social exposure or sophistication. But about 34% of the people live in urban and semi-urban areas, which are the centres of the ethnic rivalry. I suggest that these urban residents can hardly fail to share the ideological expectations of the entire Igbo. In pursuance of these expectations, the urban dwellers are likely to attempt socializing and mobilizing their compatriates at home. In this context, one would expect them to convey the biblical message: 'increase and multiply' (for therein lies our socio-economic as well as political survival) to their fellow villagers. Hence, one could argue, the politicization of the Nigerian census tends to increase fertility as well as promote population growth.

6. Educational arrangements. Although formal education was brought to Umueke as far back as 1924, it is still a scarce resource. As can be gleaned from Table 4.2, about 54% of the entire population has had no schooling at all, and another 31% has not completed primary education. Umueke is a viri-focal society, hence parents tend to give priority to male children. Consequently, literacy in Umueke is higher amongst men than women. Most of the women are thus lacking in the social exposure which education accords. They cling to the age-old spacing of children and are hardly aware of such innovations as the services of Family Planning Clinics. It must be noted that Umueke women do not share the view that population growth needs to be checked. They observe spacing only in so far as it is one of the village's post-natal rites, violation of which pollutes the social system and draws sanctions.

TABLE 4.2

Umueke's educational attainments

	Residents %	Non-residents %	Entire population %
No schooling	41	14	54
Primary not completed	20	11	31
Primary completed	4	9	12
Secondary not completed	-	0.5	1
Secondary completed	0.4	0.4	1
Post secondary	-	0.2	0.2

TABLE 4.3

Resident and non-resident females (Umueke)

Cohorts	Residents Nos.	Residents %	Non-Residents Nos.	Non-Residents %	Entire population Nos.
15 - 19	21	81	5	19	26
20 - 24	12	50	12	50	24
25 - 29	12	55	10	45	22
30 - 34	20	80	5	20	25
35 - 39	13	93	1	7	14
40 - 44	17	85	3	15	20

It must be pointed out also that Family Planning is relatively new in the East Central State, having been introduced only after the civil war (1970) by the Family Planning Council of Nigeria and the Pathfinder Fund. Moreover, the clinics are urban-based and their operations are hardly publicized in rural areas like Umueke. This helps to explain the esteem in which village herbalists like John are held, and also their role as abortionists.

7. Female non-residents. Table 4.3 indicates a fairly high incidence of out-migration amongst women. About 50% of them in the age bracket 20 - 24 and 45% in the bracket 25 - 29 are outside the village. These women are of three categories - those married into Umueke, those of Umueke origin formerly married outside the village but now divorced, and those of Umueke origin who are still single. Since the component villages of Agbaja Clan belong to the same culture-zone,[5] and Umueke men rarely recruit their wives from outside the Clan, it can be safely assumed that the three categories of women share the same fertility pattern. In normal circumstances, the trend in migration would have a delaying effect on marriage, thereby reducing fertility. But as illustrated above, most women in Umueke are illiterate and therefore are largely ill-equipped to operate effectively in the urban social and economic system. Very often those of them in the second and third categories are obliged to return home and ultimately get married. If they marry late, they make up for lost time by frequent pregnancies, with shorter than customary intervals between childbirth.

Those of the unmarried women who decide to remain in the towns are mostly obliged to become ladies of easy virtue. Since compatriots back home are largely their reference group, they hardly see any need to inhibit fertility.

8. Bridewealth. As mentioned already, bridewealth is escalating, and as a result, marriage is delayed. The delay seems to affect skilled and literate women more than it does the illiterate, who to a large extent manage to get married in their early twenties. The illiterate girls are therefore exposed to child-bearing risks for almost their total reproductive period. As for the skilled and literate women, they usually try and make up for the lost time once they get married. Hence, one could argue that the raising of the marriage age as a result of the prohibitive bridewealth has not had much impact on marital fertility.

9. Mortality rates. The discerned incidence of high fertility in Umueke has been contemporaneous with declining mortality. Life expectancy is between 40 and 42.5, and an average women has about 3.661 children and loses only .385.

---

5. Forde and Jones (1962) have delineated Igbo land into five or so culture-zones.

These statistics suggest among other things that the mortality rate is declining. It also indicates that the population is growing at a much faster rate than is suggested by the observed growth rate referred to earlier on. Three main reasons can be adduced for the declining mortality.

Firstly there has been a general improvement in environmental sanitation and cleanliness. Hygienic habits are a part of formal education. Children are now seen putting into practice habits like washing their clothes, bathing, cleaning their mouths, more often than before they went to school. They also tend to socialize their parents and mates who do not go to school in the new hygiene habits. On a more formal level, the government has taken several steps to rid the society of things that pose health hazards. For example, in 1958 the government directed that no corpse should be conveyed from one village to another. It also stipulated the time within which dead bodies must be laid to rest. These actions were prompted by a custom according to which the corpse of a widow or married woman is conveyed from her marital to her natal village for burial. Very often the funeral rites in the former location were prolonged, and the corpse started its last journey in an advanced state of decomposition, thereby exposing the society to risks of epidemics.

Second, although there exists no visible difference between the nutritive contents of food consumed by different households, such items as fish, meat, tinned food etc. are no more the rarity they were in the days of Dr. Green. There is evidence that the improved income earning capacity of the people has brought improvements in their standard of living, especially in terms of better nutrition.

Lastly, major outbreaks of smallpox and cholera have been averted by means of large scale vaccination campaigns. However, modern medical facilities are normally far removed from the village scene, which explains the people's continued reliance on herbalists like John, as well as the local drug peddlars.

Population Growth and Land

Although the area of Umueke has not been conclusively established, there are signs that the village population is increasing, pressing on limited land resources. Table 4.4 indicates that whereas 10 years ago the average fallow period in the society was 4.29 years, today it is down to only 2.71 years.

As has been illustrated earlier, Umueke is divided vertically into kin-units, the existence of which is validated by genealogies. These component lineages have tended to operate as an ideological unit in order to derive some measure of social solidarity. However, the units have also tended to develop differentially in a manner that often breeds conflict and fission in the village's social system. For example, members of one descent group may acquire more wives, bear more children and need more land. But because land is an inelastic resource, the extra land needed may be acquired at the expense of another unit. This is more so in societies that have evolved past the 'colonising' stage in Jones' (1949:310) scheme of things.

The differential expansion of the component lineages has often, over a period of time, entailed unequal individual access to land. Someone in a unit experiencing less increase in population is likely to have more land available than his counterparts in another faster growing group. But the traditional Umueke land tenure system has so far been sufficiently flexible to accommodate these changes.

The land tenure system rests on three main principles. First, the community primarily owns the land, which cannot be alienated without the members' consent. Second, access to land for the purpose of erecting a house, as well as garden and farmland cultivations, derives from membership of the patrilineage; security of tenure attaches in terms of land thus obtained. Third, no member of the lineage (and therefore the society) shall be without land. The spirit of the tenure system has been perceptively and succinctly described by Meek (1944) in the words of an Igbo elder thus:

> "Land belongs to a vast family of which many are dead, few are living and countless are still unborn."

The corporate ownership of land latently expressed by the elder makes it possible for one suffering from an acute land shortage to be 'shown land' by his compatriot who is better off. During the temporary indebtedness, a patron/client relationship never develops. The only material reward gained by the donor is a feast given by the beneficiary which usually costs no more than £2.50.

In spite of the land tenure system's orientation towards corporate holding, individual ownership is beginning to feature. This is due largely to such factors as inheritance and differential numerical growth. In terms of individual ownership, a man could relinquish his title over his land temporarily, as when he 'shows' land. He could also abandon his title permanently when he passes the land on to his son or relation. Outright sale of land is strictly prohibited and draws grave sanctions. The society conceives of land as the resting place of the ancestors, and therefore something sacred which must not be defiled and disposed of like other chattels in the market. Hence although land fragmentation is occurring, speculation and consolidation are hardly featuring. One can therefore sum up the rationale behind the land tenure system as: 'Not free for all but fair for all'. The vested interest in continuing succession to land reinforces the stress placed on high fertility in Umueke and the consequent condemnation of abortions.

TABLE 4.4

Comparative analysis of fallow period and changes in land ownership

	Mean average 1975 (years)	Mean average 1965 (years)	Percentage of decrease	% of those whose land has increased over the 10 years	% of those whose land has decreased over the 10 years	% of those whose land has remained the same over the 10 years
Entire Society	2.71	4.29	37	41	18	41
Top Stratum	2.50	3.50	40	50	25	25
Second Stratum	2.75	5.25	100	75	25	-
Third Stratum	3.00	4.25	42	50	-	50
Bottom Stratum	2.60	4.20	62	-	20	80

Agricultural Potential and Migration

In spite of the persistence of shifting cultivation in Umueke,[6] the society experiences a comparatively high incidence of out-migration. As noted before, about 34% of the entire population lives outside the village. The high incidence of out-migration can be attributed to the society's demographic trends as much as it can be said to derive from the comparative advantages urban life offers. Since the mid-forties or so, successive governments of Nigeria have evolved quinquennial policies for the nation's socio-economic as well as political advancement. These policies, officially designated National Development Plans, have been very urban-oriented. Moreover, there has been a chasm between the objectives of the Plans and the implementation.

As a result Umueke, like other constituent villages of Agbaja, lacks infra-structural facilities. The nearest tarred road is the Enugu-Umuahia Trunk A which is about 10 miles away. The road cuts Mbano into two, leaving Agbaja in the southern half. Umueke is linked to the road by three barely motorable roads, as well as several bush paths. These outlets are marshy in the rainy season and dusty in the dry season. The village lacks electricity and pipe-borne water. Even Mbano, the Division Headquarters, lacks these facilities. Although Western education was first introduced in Umueke about 51 years ago, there are today only eight or so strategically located primary schools serving the entire Agbaja area. The Clan's first secondary school is in the process of being established only as a result of the joint efforts of the Community Council and the various chapters of the urban-based 'Town Union'.[7] As mentioned already, the village also lacks modern medical facilities like maternity clinics and hospitals.

Thus isolated and lacking in basic amenities, Umueke is a very rural society. The village's employment structure, as gleaned from Table 4.5, indicates that farming is the people's dominant occupation. Table 4.6 illustrates Umueke's cash earnings and reveals that farming is also the mainstay of the society's economy. The chief cash crop is the oil palm.

---

6. That Umueke is not really in distress in terms of land resources is further evidenced by the facts:

   (a) that up till now, the people have not felt the need to register their respective pieces of land;

   (b) that a search through court records did not reveal any land litigation involving the villagers;

   (c) informants could not remember any dispute.

7. A Town Union is a mutual aid social organisation formed to cater for the interest of members of a corporate group resident in an urban or semi-urban centre.

TABLE 4.5

Resident population's employment structure

Occupation	Percentage of population
Farmers	66
Casual labourers	13
Trado-medics (herbalists/diviners)	13
Petty traders	4
Teachers	2
Clerk typist (working for the government)	1
Bike repairer	1
Total	100

TABLE 4.6

Umueke's annual cash earnings

Source	Percentage of total earnings
Palm wine)	
Palm oil)	45
Palm kernel)	
Food crop)	
Casual labour)	36
Salaried labour)	
Petty trading (excludes farm produce)	5
Contributions	4
Money received from children or husbands	4
Rents collected from machines & houses	2
Bike repairing	4
Total	100

Processing palm nuts at the oil-pressing machine is a joint endeavour involving the man of the family, his wife/wives, and at times his mother and unmarried sisters. Since the palm is a man's crop, he retains the proceeds from the sale of palm-oil. Those accruing from such by-products as the kernel go to all the women who helped in pressing the oil.

The principal staple crops are: yam, cassava, co-co yam, maize, beans, okro, ground-nuts, pepper, broad-leaf pumpkin, fluted pumpkin, and many other types of vegetable. The nuclear family, or the household[8] in the case of a polygynous family, is the unit of production. That is to say, labour is drawn largely from a man's wife/wives and child/children. However, it is not unusual for a man to be supplied with labour by his friends or age (youth) mates on reciprocal terms. Wage labour is the rare exception; the only paid agricultural labour is that hired to cut down ripe oil palm nuts.

There is considerable division of labour according to sex and age. For example, clearing the bush and making mounds are deemed a man's job, while weeding and conveying harvested crops home are the lot of women and children respectively. In spite of the fact that cassava has overtaken yam in importance, the former continues to be regarded as a woman's crop while the latter is considered a man's responsibility. Umueke's agricultural system has been constrained by such factors as very low technological inputs, poor soil fertility,[9] the people's unwillingness to organise co-operatives etc. With the exception of the recently acquired domesticated oil-palm seedlings belonging to the incumbent village Councillor, high yielding varieties are not in use in the village. Moreover, other new technologies such as chemical fertilizers, pesticides, herbicides, relevant machinery etc., are not utilised. It is pertinent to note that most heads of households have indicated their unwillingness to participate in co-operative farming. This is perhaps a manifestation of the individualised competitiveness of the Igbo.

In the thirteen or so months in which I lived in Umueke, no extension officer called. Yet there was an Agricultural Extension Office only 8 miles away. When asked why they were not availing themselves of the innovations provided by the Extension Office, the villagers answered invariably that some of the so-called innovations are 'too artificial', that crops grown with fertilizers do not preserve well, that the cost of the

---

8. In delineating a household, I have used the criterion of eating from the same pot. The Igbo equivalent is *'Akwukwa'*.
9. The soils of Umueke are very stony, and like most tropical soils, are deficient in calcium and other plant nutrients due largely to the leaching actions of torrential rainfalls. The rains often wash away the necessary plant food and minerals contained in the top layer of the soils, and also cause gully erosion.

inputs advised by the Extension Officers is rather prohibitive. Some farmers also felt neglected and slighted by the officers. The officers, for their part, alleged that most of the farmers are very culture bound and simply would not respond to innovative overtures.

There are some elements of truth on both sides. The farmers are largely illiterate, which therefore tends to make them more tradition-oriented and averse to innovations. On the other hand, the Extension Office was virtually empty. It received - at irregular intervals - a rather token supply of fertilizer, high-yielding varieties and other such new technologies. This is somewhat curious considering Nigeria's huge budgetary allocations to agriculture. It is even more surprising that the minimal supply which reached the Extension Office was often salted away and eventually sold to farmers elsewhere near urban areas, who are engaged in cash cropping. The communication gap between Umueke farmers and the agricultural officers makes it mandatory that the extension services should be re-organised.

The largely primitive and seemingly static agricultural system of Umueke appears to be finding it increasingly difficult to sustain the fast growing population of the village. True, the villagers still sell some of their food crops, especially at harvest time. This is done partly to obtain the much-needed cash for meeting expenses like school fees, and partly due to the fact that the crops might go bad, since storage poses enormous problems. Many have to buy more food during slack periods.

The high incidence of out-migration in Umueke has considerably exacerbated the village's agricultural problems. It has been shown that about twice as many people in the active age bracket 19-39 live outside the village than within it. The degree of out-migration therefore poses another serious problem: food production is left in the hands of weaker and older people. This tends to affect adversely the efficiency of the production system, and reduces both per capita and per acre output. The high level of out-migration also creates dependency problems, since the migrants often join urban populations which are agriculturally dependent on the rural sector.

The supervening crisis in Umueke's food production system has itself contributed immensely to the society's relatively high rate of migration. As farming becomes increasingly less remunerative, the villagers are obliged to explore alternative avenues for achieving upward social mobility. Out-migration is one of the options open to them; it enables the migrant to do wage labour and earn cash, part of which he invariably remits to the village. Thus out-migration makes it possible for the society to link its surplus labour force with the wider national labour market.

However despite the benefits, out-migration aggravates the food production problems of Umueke, thereby contributing to poverty in the society.

Umueke's poverty is a multi-dimensional phenomenon. When viewed in absolute terms it manifests itself in the general condition prevailing in the village of: *low income*, as a result of unemployment and diminishing agricultural out-put per capita, as well as per acre; *poor health*, deriving from lack of modern medical facilities, and inadequate adoption of proper hygiene habits; *malnutrition*, due to unbalanced diet; *low literacy rate*, stemming from lack of educational facilites. On the other hand, when the poverty situation is considered in relative terms, the overriding determinants are seen to be the human and spatial developmental imbalances. Such disparities in material growth can be induced and perpetuated, as has been illustrated, by differential population growth, prolonged attachment to out-moded cultural values, or biased socio-economic advancement policies. These variables act cumulatively to make the rich richer and the poor poorer. Moreover, they tend to result in the development of the urban centres largely at the expense of such rural areas a Umueke.

Migration and Village Membership

Peter Elemai, the 'Regent' who acts for John Obioma, the 'Crown Prince', exemplifies the costs and benefits of out-migration. Peter lived in the Cameroons for 32 years, during which time he traded and did various wage jobs.

As far as Umueke is concerned, migration is not conceived on a permanent basis because membership of the patrilineage is eternal. Moreover, the city lacks that village flavour which tends to make everybody his brother's keeper and provides security for all. Hence, although the city holds out more job and income opportunities than the village, it is too dehumanised for the liking of the Umueke migrant. One such migrant referred to city life as *'Ike keta orie'*, i.e. 'survival of the fittest'. The vagaries of urban life motivate migrants from rural areas to keep in touch with their home base, so that if necessary they can always return and be readily absorbed in the village. Uchendu (1965:34) aptly commented:

> "Almost from the start the individual is aware of his dependence on his kin group and his community ... It is his ultimate desire to return to his village after earning money elsewhere. To him, the village is the appropriate place for retirement, the city a place to earn money."

Membership of the lineage, like most social relationships, attracts duties, obligations and rights. In Umueke and most Igbo villages a 'mass return' of non-resident (migrant) members is ordered almost every year at such traditional occasions as the 'new-yam' festival, or at such Christian festivities as Christmas. Failure to comply with the come-home order often draws sanctions. The mass return serves two main purposes. First it enables the society to collect levies from all citizens for providing social amenities within the framework of community development. Second, it also affords the migrants the opportunity of re-affirming their membership of the society. Moreover, it serves the residual function of abating conflicts, since such a home-coming could help pre-empt attempts by residents to violate the rights of non-residents. One such infringment of the right of a non-resident is evidenced in the case of Ben Igwe, who has four wives and ten children[10] when he encroached on a piece of land owned by Obi Okoye, who belongs to the same lineage as Ben. The latter's children are mostly boys, and so finding enough land for them is quite problematic. Ben, in fact, is short of land. Obi, on the other hand, has only one wife and three children (two boys and one girl), and unlike Ben, he has more land than he actually needs. Ben's intrusion into Obi's land was facilitated only by the latter's long absence from the village. His stint on the plantation of the Cameroons lasted for fourteen almost uninterrupted years. Members of the lineage did not act to stop Ben's intrusion, probably because of the break in communication with Obi. Moreover, the Igbo say: *"Ada edebelu onye jelu Asaba anu okuku"* i.e. "you don't reserve chicken meat for someone who is not around to claim his own share".

At the same time out-migration may lead to upward social mobility. For instance, Peter the 'Regent' now has two wives, six children and one of the eight comparatively modern houses in the village. While operating in the urban social milieu of the Cameroons, he seemed to have internalized the trait of delayed gratification, which is hardly an attribute of his natal society. He invested part of his relatively higher income in two buildings at Obigbo, the town to which most of his compatriots go for seasonal wage labour. He now lives off the rent accruing from these houses. He supplements this income by practising trado-medicalism (herbalism), which ranks high in the income structure of the village. Peter now finds it convenient to rely less on agricultural income, which as has been illustrated, is becoming increasingly precarious. In Umueke, where there is no institutionalised mode of signifying affluence, such as taking a title, Peter plays his wealth down. But with a conservatively estimated annual income of about £140 in a society where many earn only £2 per annum, Peter is certainly one of the richest in the village.

Incest and Abortion

Having sketched in the background to the abortion case, it is now possible to analyse some of its major features.

The sorrowing silence that immediately pervaded the village

---

10. One of the children is actually an illegitimate son of Ben's fourth wife. Ben is not the child's biological father. But since he acquired the son together with his mother at marriage, the child now has an equal right to inherit Ben's property like his other legitimate children. Moreover, the adopted child is now fully integrated into the patrilineage.

denotes how appalled and alienated the people felt. The reaction stems from the fact that there is a rule which prescribes that all redresses should be sought in the first instance within the traditional judicial framework. This rule is a measure of the people's protectionism, as well as their parochial political culture. The orientation towards the traditional judicial process is legitimised at intervals by villagers being directed to swear oaths. They swear that all disputes, both criminal and civil, must be brought before the village tribunal before they are referred to the Common Law Courts. The role played by the Ikpeamas, who defied both the oath and the rule, suggests, *prima facie*, the breaking down of the society's norms. The apparently waning influence of the norms derives largely from the diffusion of urban values into the village's social system. Umueke villagers thought that the redress sought by the Ikpeamas was the brain child of one Gab Ikpeama, who resides and does wage labour at Obigbo.

Gab is the maternal uncle of Ahudie. He is also literate, and in the somewhat pluralistic setting of Obigbo he seems to have adopted some impersonal and contractual norms. It is likely that these norms motivated him to advise his compound to seek Common Law redress. Gab appeared more concerned with the abortion aspect of the case, which was a criminal offence, than with John's presumed violation of the village's incest taboo. Thus Gab's role entailed identification with the wider society, as well as a perceived attempt to diffuse an alien pattern of behaviour into the traditional social system. Though it may be an oversimplification, it appears that his identification with the wider society was indirectly prompted by population growth, which with other contributory factors necessitated the out-migration that improved his financial status. It was his position as one of the 'nouveau riche' which enabled him to opt for the Common Law redress. He paid as much as £75 to brief Counsel to defend Ahudie, who was charged as an accomplice. This fee, which far out-strips the cost of litigation within the traditional framework, is a great deal in terms of the average per capita income in Umueke.

Since the end of the court case the Ikpeamas seem to be suffering from a guilt complex, and there have been whispers that the traditional machinery of justice will be set in motion. It is being suggested that the Ikpeamas will be requested by the entire village to substantiate their allegations on a sasswood oath, and John will similarly have to affirm his innocence. It is also being rumoured that, come what may, sanctions will be exerted on the Ikpeamas for manoeuvring outside the traditional scheme of things.

If the Ikpeamas swear to the oath and bear the sanctions, the society will have resolved the supervening crisis and restored equilibrium to the social system. If, on the other hand, they refuse to take the restorative steps, there are two possible alternatives. The society will either have to accommodate them or ostracise them until performance of the acts. Either way, the crisis will persist with a precedent having been set for further defiance of the society's rules.

In spite of the fact that the court has handed down a not-guilty verdict, there seems to be a lurking suspicion that John committed the acts alleged by the Ikpeamas. If his guilt is established on an oath, he will have broken two oaths - one in respect of incest and the other regarding homicide. The contravention is bound to draw sanctions despite his eminence. A saying goes: *'Igbo enwe eze'* meaning 'The Igbos do not have kings'. It symbolises many social realities. It connotes the egalitarian ethos of the Igbo, and also explains to some extent their decentralised political system. Above all, it conceptualises the people's notion of 'The Rule of Law', which emphasises that nobody is above the law of the society.

Umueke is a corporate group as well as an exogamous unit. It is to effect compliance with the rules of exogamy that the oath referred to above is administered in order to prevent incest. One of the crucial factors determining the degree of compliance with such an oath is the trend in the society's demography. In a closed society experiencing a negative growth rate there is likely to be the need for component lineages to coalesce. This trend towards fusion is also likely to prompt manipulation of genealogies to justify the realignments. It will above all generate pressure to observe incest rules.

On the other hand, in a society like Umueke experiencing a fairly high fertility rate, the trend in inter-lineage relations is more likely to be fission and accretion. This tends to expand the social distance between classificatory brothers and sisters, and increases the temptation to commit incest, thereby breaking the rules of exogamy. Moreover, population growth, as we have noted, induces out-migration and the diffusion of urban values into the rural social system. These urban norms are necessarily impersonal, and tend to weaken the spirit of 'togetherness' between villagers, especially amongst the youngsters.

Incest occurs frequently in Umueke, but it draws no sanctions until pregnancy results. The last cleansing ceremony was performed in the village in 1958. Incidentally, Ahudie herself is the product of an incestuous relationship. In her parents' case, although there may have been attempts at abortion, the society laid no emphasis on this but was more concerned with the incestuous aspect of the episode. This contrasts strongly with the John/Ahudie case, where the normative sanctions they incurred were the result of the abortion rather than the fact of incest.

Umueke's moral condemnation of homicide of any kind (including abortion) is perhaps best rationalised thus: 'Do not take any human life since you cannot restore it'. And the ideals of the ban are most succinctly expressed in the saying: *'Onye ma Echi'* i.e. 'Who knows tomorrow (what the expected child will grow to be)?'. The discouragement of abortion can also be interpreted in terms of the people's tendency towards large families. However, in spite of the oath, there seem to be many more instances of abortion than the two narrated to me.

Earlier I indicated the high incidence of incest in Umueke. Such incestuous relations are likely to result in pregnancies which the women involved wish to terminate by abortions. Umueke women are hardly aware of any other means of family planning, apart from practising the traditional spacing. They are therefore prone to a high incidence of pregnancy. This explains to some extent the relatively high fertility rate. If the unwanted pregnancy is not terminated the unmarried mother could be condemned to perpetual spinsterhood. Alternatively the bride-wealth that will be paid for her later when she gets married could be very small, as was the case with Ben Igwe's fourth wife, who had an illegitimate child. Since there is no hospital or maternity clinic to offer contraceptive advice, the burden of effecting abortion and giving information about it falls on John and his seven herbalist colleagues. Fearing the consequences of admitting to having committed a criminal offence, they talk (if at all) about their operations in the context of 'Do not say I said'. Some of the abortions may well be effected far away from the surveying eyes of the society. In the circumstances, problems involved in attempting to quantify the clandestine efforts defy imagination.

Pregnancy occurring within the spacing period is as bad as that resulting from incest. Both precipitate a state of social dysphoria and necessitate a purification of the social system. As in the case of incest, it is not a pleasant experience to carry out a cleansing rite. So when pregnancy occurs within the stipulated spacing period, the offending couple are likely to seek a clandestine abortion. Hence, as mentioned earlier on, the frequency of abortion in Umueke is higher than the observed incidents suggest.

Political Office and Social Status

In accordance with custom, the Ikpeamas should have lodged their complaint with the head of their major lineage, i.e. Peter the 'Regent' or the village Councillor, Bob Osuji. The Ikpeamas may have felt justified in suspecting that they would not have obtained justice from Peter, who is John's uncle. The proximity of the relationship between the two made the complainants suspect that the former might have a vested interest in the dispute, and it is certainly equitable that no one should be an arbiter in a matter to which he is a party. Granting that, one still wonders why they did not alternatively complain to the Councillor, who to all intents and purposes is sufficiently detached.

Here Bob's lowly social status as an *'Umeh'* may offer a clue. In spite of several Christian as well as legislative efforts, Umueke still operates a caste system which ascribes a superior status to the free-born *'Amadi'* and inferior status to the cult-slave *'Osuh'* and the members of a jinxed family *'Umeh'*. There are about 58 *Osuhs* and 30 *Umehs* in Umueke, and they constitute about 16% of the entire population. The caste system is comparatively liberal. True, Umueke society does not accord their low castes much respectability; they are precluded from traditional government and are forbidden to break the Kola for the free-born. But they do enjoy equal access to land and other means of production, and are fully integrated economically as well as in terms of modern leadership.

Making a living in Umueke is inextricably tied up with the land, and since land use and rights are open to all Bob has shrewdly maintained a large family work force with a view to optimising his agricultural output. The economies of scale entailed in his acquiring two wives and producing ten children, and the accruing benefits, suggests a material justification for Umueke's ban on abortion. Although there is a low conceptual stress on the utility of, and output from, child labour, Bob seems to owe a lot to his children in terms of his relative affluence. His first daughter, Joy, who is still unmarried at twenty, helps out in farm work as well as in pressing her father's palm oil. She also trades and makes a considerable profit. Bob has many such industrious children, and hopes 'to go on making more babies'.

Thanks to the joint efforts of the family, Bob has been able to see his first son, Jimmy, through a secondary education. Western education, as noted earlier, is still a scarce resource in the village due to the high rate of illiteracy. Hence investment in education often brings high rewards. Today, Jimmy is gainfully employed at Sapele, and he sends an undisclosed amount home regularly to help train his younger brother in school.

Bob himself is one of the few elder citizens who are literate. The villagers believe that the interaction between Umueke and the wider state or national polity necessitates sophisticated leadership. It is in recognition of Bob's relative education and affluence that his lineage has nominated him as the village Councillor. The office rotates between the four major lineages which constitute the village. A Councillor holds office for two years.

Bob occupies Umueke's main modern leadership role by virtue of the fact that he liaises between the village and a wider polity. He sits in the Agbaja Umukabia Community Council - a local authority - with other Councillors representing the various corporate groups in the clan area. Thus each of the constituent villages represents a ward of the Council. The Council acts as an intermediary between the clan's people and the State Government.

As a Councillor, Bob convenes village meetings and communicates Council decisions to the assembly. He executes such decisions as collection of Capitation Tax or other levies imposed for Community development. He also conveys the wishes of his villagers to the Council. Bob adjudicates over village disputes and is expected to sign bail bonds for arrested villagers. Although constitutional authority resides with the Community Council, the real power to effect Community development and modernisation of the social system seems to lie with the several chapters of Umueke Progressive Union. The chapters are largely urban-based, and collectively appear to command more resources and personalities than the Council. Hence it is also Bob's duty to establish rapport with the Unions with a view to co-ordinating their efforts with those of the Council and the 'Progressive Unions' of other constituent villages.

Although Umueke stresses an egalitarian ethos and discourages political or economic dominance of one individual by another, Bob has been trying to lay the foundation for future dominance. As a measure of his relative affluence noted earlier, he owns one of the three oil-pressing machines in the village. Moreover, he strives to augment his wealth by all means, fair or foul. Thus he draws resentment from his compatriots, especially the indolent ones. Since his appointment as Councillor, Bob has exhibited some surprising venality. He has been using his office as a source of unofficial profit. He accepts bribes for doing his normal duties, and has been able to acquire high-yielding palm seedlings - the first of their kind in the village.

The feeling of resentment which Bob attracts appears to be a protest against the ambitious economic manipulations of an upstart who is abusing the leadership role assigned to him. The somewhat philistine image which Bob has cut for himself, and the supervening crises of confidence which the image has prompted, make the villagers wonder if their experimental liberalism - which facilitated the admission of a low caste member to the society's modern leadership - should continue. The somewhat hypersensitive stance of the villagers is a reflection of the paternalism and anti-individualism which is inherent in the social system. Similarly the Ikpeamas approach to the Courts rather than to their village Councillor can be taken as a symbol of the free-born's contempt for a low-caste upstart.

Conclusion

By means of the extended case method (Van Velsen, 1967:129), I have attempted in this paper to discuss the inter-relationship between various economic, political and social factors, and their impact on the demographic processes of Umueke. This interdependence is clearly reflected in the social norms relating to abortion, incest and birth-spacing in the village, the belief in reincarnation, reinforced by the economic advantages derived from large numbers of wives and children, and the stress on tribal ethnicity which in Nigeria's political system emphasises the need for growing numbers of voters, and which accounts to some extent for the strong resistance against abortion.

The extended case method has perhaps thrown up some seeming contradictions in Umueke's social system. In spite of the already adduced reasons, one might still wonder why the people continue to strive for large families, thereby increasing their population in the face of their very precarious economy, characterised by dwindling natural resources and very low technology. Another question could also arise as to why the people still prefer male children to females, even though the former present many problems in terms of allocating sufficient land, and even though the latter bring in considerable income through bridewealth.

These posers - and others of their kind - manifest the problem involved in looking at simple societies like Umueke from a material point of view only. To all intents and purposes this somewhat one-dimensional perspective fails to grasp fully the internal logic of such social systems, since it plays down or even ignores the spiritual factor in the roles played in such societies. This spiritual flavour is well brought out in the Igbo name: *'Azu ka ego'*, meaning that ensuring a man's posterity and the perpetuation of the patrilineage is more gainful than amassing wealth. This manifestation of the Umueke *Weltanschauung* may help to explain some of the apparent paradoxes.

CHART 4.1

UMUEKE 1974: AGE/SEX PYRAMID - RESIDENT POPULATION

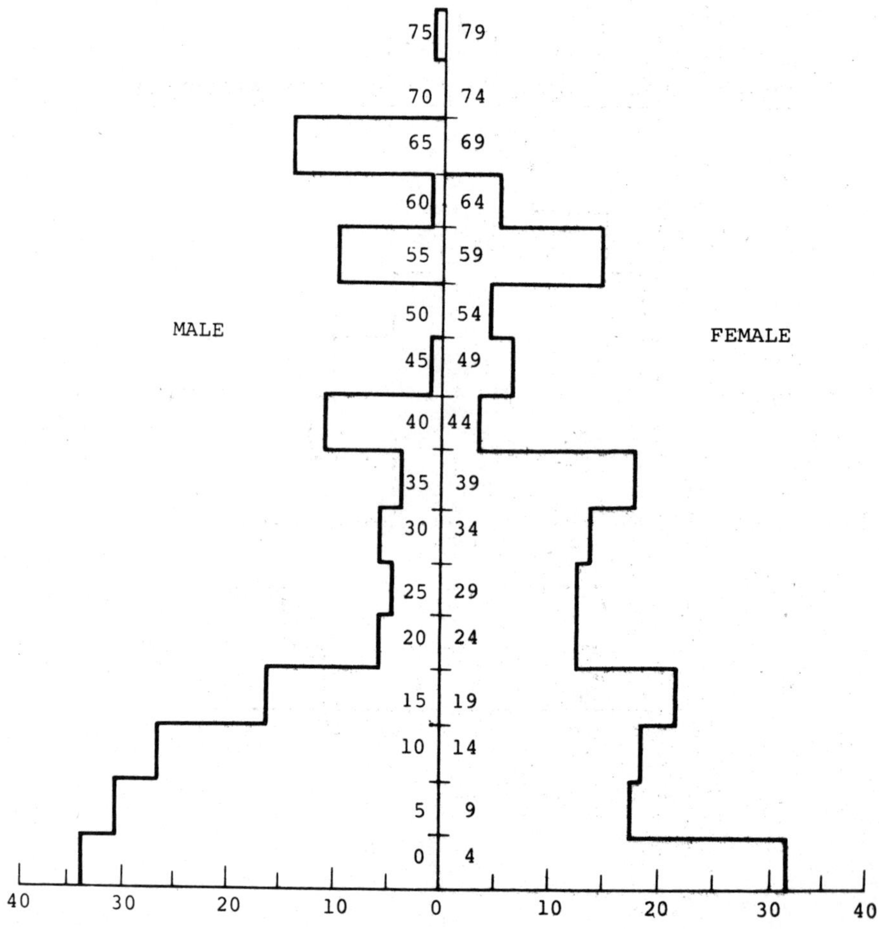

CHART 4.2

UMUEKE 1974: AGE/SEX PYRAMID - NON-RESIDENTS

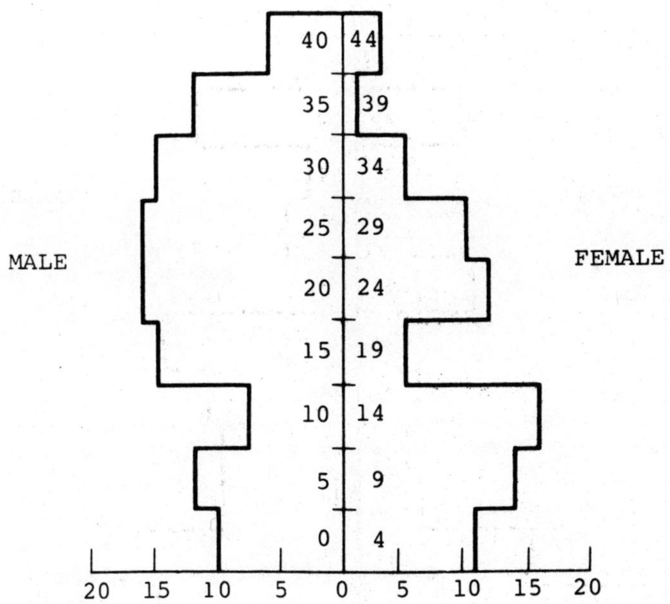

CHAPTER 5

FROM A CLOSED TO AN OPEN SYSTEM: FERTILITY BEHAVIOUR IN A CHANGING INDIAN VILLAGE

INTRODUCTION

In the past few years, there has been a growing interest amongst demographers and others in studying the relationship between the level of fertility and the socio-economic context in which it takes place. This may have arisen from dissatisfaction with current macro-explanations of fertility differentials and changes. These theories, which try to encompass all observations at once, concentrate attention on the *presence* of the explanatory variables used in a situation of fertility decline, rather than on the *mechanisms* whereby they affect fertility.[1]

The theory of the demographic transition describes the process in which mortality decline is followed by fertility decline, with an intermediate period of relatively rapid population growth. The transition is found to correspond with the 'industrialization' or 'modernization' (the two concepts often being used interchangeably) of a society, and with increased levels of education, as well as a number of other variables mostly associated with 'modernization'. Although one of the originators of the theory, Notestein, stated that only the general validity of the theory had been proven and that what was needed was knowledge at lower levels of generality, little work has been done on this latter aspect.

As a result there is a strong tendency to conceive of 'modernization' and 'education' as forces which, in an almost mystical way, change the fertility behaviour of a society. From this, one might be led to hypothesize a fairly straightforward correlation between variations in the level of, e.g. education, and parity. Coale (1973) highlighted the problems involved in such an approach after conducting a highly detailed study of the correlates of fertility decline in every region of Europe.

Thus he says 'Essentially, universal primary education had been achieved in Germany and Scandinavia by 1870 but fertility there remained on a high plateau'. Elsewhere in that paper, he lists three conditions[2] for fertility decline and says 'Apparently modernization establishes these three conditions, but also,

---

1. This problem has been discussed, e.g. by Robert Cassen in his forthcoming book on population and development in India.
2. Briefly, these are: acceptance of calculated choice in fertility; perception of advantages of reduced fertility; knowledge and mastery of effective contraceptive techniques.

apparently, they can occur in little modernized communities'. Many papers have been written on the correlation between education and fertility, but there are hardly any studies which attempt to establish why such a relationship exists.

Another aspect of demographic transition theory is that it has been noticed for a long time that fertility decline in many European and other societies began in the upper or middle classes, but one of the few attempts to explain why this should be so has been made by Banks (1954), who showed that it was the middle classes who started the fertility decline in England in the late nineteenth century. He argues that, given aspirations for a high standard of living both for themselves and for their children, and faced with the rising costs of bringing up and educating children in the ways considered necessary, the English middle classes could no longer afford high fertility.

Perhaps in an attempt to turn away from this macro-level approach, there has been a recent growth of interest in cost/benefit analyses of childbearing. Leaving aside considerations as to whether or not such analyses are really feasible, this approach has the defect of being too highly individual-oriented. Individuals do not necessarily make decisions about their fertility behaviour in any very precisely calculated way. Yet clearly there is an overall correspondence between the fertility behaviour of a population and the economic opportunities open to them. It is important to remember that people have always known how to control their fertility through abortion, infanticide and delayed marriage[3] but these methods are on the whole not satisfactory. Also it is unlikely that their use without modern contraception or safe simple means of abortion would keep fertility low in the face of the dramatic modern declines in mortality. For example, the decline in fertility commonly associated with a shift from a peasant to an industrialized economy must be largely due to the change in the costs and advantages of childbearing involved. Those peasant societies which have reduced their fertility seem to be those in which their main source of subsistence - land - is becoming rapidly fragmented.[4]

Any attempt to remedy the deficiencies inherent in the two approaches outlined above demands an alternative method of understanding fertility behaviour. The analytical gap between the

---

3. Notestein (1953), pointed out that the fertility decline in many European societies was achieved by methods long known but unused until the incentive for birth control increased.
4. Demeny's (1972) work on Austro-Hungary shows pockets of declining fertility in the rural areas with infant mortality very high in comparison with present day underdeveloped countries. He says that there was even a trend towards raising only one child, and suggests as an explanation a desire to avoid fragmentation of landholdings. In the mid-nineteenth century the Irish reduced their fertility for similar reasons.

macro and the cost/benefit approach may be bridged by concentrating on the *mechanisms* through which fertility behaviour is influenced by the economic environment. To a large extent the behaviour of individuals is guided by the norms of the group to which they belong. These group norms constitute the intervening variable, since they are in turn influenced by the economic environment. Thus:-

```
Economic environment
    |           |
    v           |
Group norms     |
    |           |
    v           v
Individual fertility behaviour
```

This conceptualization is clearly over-simplistic, since each of the three factors represents only a part of the total reality. Fertility behaviour is affected by a wide variety of non-economic factors, such as religious beliefs, the psychic benefits of childbearing and so on. If it can be shown that most of these other factors influence all groups of a society, to a greater or lesser extent, and only their economic situation and fertility appear to vary significantly, then there is reason to conclude that economic factors are the major ones affecting fertility.

In this paper I attempt to go beyond observing the mere coexistence of 'modernization' variables on the one hand and fertility decline on the other. I try to analyse the *mechanisms* which may account for these phenomena. I base my examination on data I collected in Rampur, a village 15 miles from Delhi, which was first studied by Oscar Lewis in 1953.[5]

I argue that, given the nature of certain changes within the village and the wider economy, the risks and uncertainties inherent in a society with subsistence agriculture and high mortality rates have been considerably diminished. The villagers can manipulate more accurately the various options open to them and carry them out with a greater degree of certainty about likely implications and consequences. In this sense their control over their environment has increased correspondingly. Moreover, I argue that the nature of these new options requires heavy investment in terms of time and money and hence puts a premium on low fertility. This contrasts with the situation in the traditional society, in which high fertility was of possible economic value.

Thus the decline in fertility which has so often been seen as coinciding roughly with the transition from a peasant to an industrialized economy can be explained, certainly in the context of this particular village, in terms of the strategies for best exploiting the options open to people in these two types of economy.

---

5. Lewis, O. (1958), *Village Life in Northern India*, University of Illinois Press, Urbana.

TABLE 5.1

Land distribution by caste, 1975

Caste	Landless		Less than 5 Bighas*		5 - 10 Bighas		10 - 20 Bighas		20 - 50 Bighas		50+ Bighas		Total	
	No.	%	No.	%	No.	%	No.	%	No.	%	No.	%	No.	%
Jat	-	-	8	6.2	21	16.2	35	27.2	44	34.2	21	16.2	129**	100
Brahmins	-	-	4	19.0	5	23.8	11	52.3	1	4.7	-	-	21	100
Chamars	29	96.7	1	3.3	-	-	-	-	-	-	-	-	30	100
Bhangis	16	100	-	-	-	-	-	-	-	-	-	-	16	100
Jhimmars	13	100	-	-	-	-	-	-	-	-	-	-	13	100
Nai, Badai, Chippi, Baniya	16	84.3	-	-	3	15.7	-	-	-	-	-	-	19	100
Lohar, Kumhar, Dhobi	13	100	-	-	-	-	-	-	-	-	-	-	13	100

* 4.8 bighas = 1 acre (approx.)

** The difference between total number of Jat households and families (see Table 5.3) is accounted for by several families owning and operating land jointly.

In view of the fact that the fieldwork is still in progress, the hypotheses put forward in this chapter are only tentative, but it should be added that the villagers' own description of their situation lends support to my argument.

The Historical Background of Rampur

Rampur is situated 15 miles west of Delhi, historically within Punjab/Haryana. This region has for long been one of the most affluent in India, and was used by the British as a source of foodgrain for famine-struck districts. The area has been canal-irrigated since the turn of the century. There was low population pressure, due to the opening up of vast new tracts of land on the western side by digging canals. Population was then transferred to these newly irrigated areas. Darling (1957) estimates that, until 1921, the land under cultivation increased considerably relative to the population, and that this process was reversed only between 1921-1931. Thus till 1921-1931, the region had every reason to expand population fast, in order to fully exploit the newly cultivable land.[6]

In the relatively short period of time - approximately three decades - which followed, the situation has changed completely, with a sudden burst of population growth (see Appendix 5.1). Large numbers of people are being pushed off the land, and so there is every incentive to control fertility.

Another important feature of the region is that landholding is fairly evenly distributed (see Table 5. 1) in comparison with other parts of India. The value of the land and the price of agricultural produce rose considerably,[7] especially with the two World Wars. Thus there was already considerable accumulation of wealth in the rural area, so that the expensive new agricultural technology was taken up as soon as it became available.

After Independence in 1947, there was a rapid growth in the Administration and thus in tertiary sector jobs. This situation was exploited by those who had a certain amount of education at the time, and this has now had a demonstration effect on the rest of the population, who see that these office jobs are relatively undemanding and well paid. Since the Delhi area is fairly industrialized, a variety of jobs are potentially open to the villagers.

In 1953, when the village was studied by Oscar Lewis, only a few people were earning outside incomes (see Table 5.2), but on the whole the village economy absorbed most of the population. Agriculture was primarily for subsistence purposes, and most of

---

6. As Darling points out, this was indeed the case: the richest districts had the highest rates of natural increase.
7. Darling mentions that by 1921, irrigated land in some areas cost more than good land in Britain.

TABLE 5.2

Distribution of urban occupations by caste, 1953

Total No. of men age 15-64	Caste	Army/ Police	Teachers	Factory workers, clerks and transport	Low jobs*
203	Jats	15	12	25	
28	Brahmins	8	5	7	2
28	Chamars				4
15	Bhangis				2
42	Kumhar				2
42	Nai		1		
42	Badai		2		

* Peons etc.

TABLE 5.3

Fragmentation of Jat land-holdings (1953 - 1975)

	Less than 5 bighas*		5 - 20 bighas		20 - 50 bighas		50 - 100 bighas		100 - 200 bighas		200+ bighas	
	No.	%	No.	%	No.	%	No.	%	No.	%	No.	%
1953*	3	3.8	22	28.2	29	37.1	17	21.7	6	7.6	1	1.2
1975	8	6.2	56	43.4	44	34.1	18	13.9	3	2.3	-	

* Details in Lewis's table (p.102) are given in acreages which have been converted here at the rate of one acre for five bighas.

the village population managed to live off the land, either directly or indirectly. The landowning castes and the service castes formed an organic unit, at least as far as production was concerned. The service castes, who are mostly landless in Rampur, were paid in kind for their labour and took in plots for cultivation on a fixed money rent basis. Those Jats who had additional small landholdings had little difficulty in acquiring land for sharecropping.

Between 1953 and 1975, many changes have taken place in the village. Agriculture has been revolutionized. A Primary Health Centre and several more schools have been built in the vicinity. In the late 1960's, electricity was brought in and a proper road built connecting Rampur directly with Delhi. Bus services have been constantly improving and are now frequent and regular. Rampur has been in a very advantageous position as a result of being part of Delhi Union Territory for administrative purposes, and has thus reaped the benefits of considerable infrastructural investments.[8]

Broadly speaking there have been three important consequences of this recent period of change: the village has become closely integrated with the wider economy; there has been a shift in agriculture from being primarily subsistence-oriented to cash cropping; and a large proportion of households are now dependent on outside income.

Changes in the Agricultural Sphere 1953-1975

The new agricultural technology was adopted during the 1960's. This included tractors,[9] tubewells, chemical fertilizers, and high-yielding varieties of seed. These new techniques are now being applied to almost all the land.[10] Output per crop increased considerably. There has been a shift from single cropping to double and triple cropping, since tractors make it possible to prepare land quickly after the harvest for the next crop.

Two forces are operating which make for the dislocation of labour from agriculture. One is mechanization, which means that the heaviest operations are now done by tractor and tubewell, (i.e. ploughing and threshing). The other factor is the growth of population and the consequent division of landholdings (see

8. These infra-structural elements have also been established in the state of Haryana, where the excellent rural transport services bring commuters daily to the great number of small urban centres.

9. There are 13 tractors in the village, and others in neighbouring villages, so there is rarely any shortage of tractors for those who want to hire them. A small proportion of the village land is not under tubewell irrigation. A few families still use oxen instead of tractors.

10. The man-land ratio has doubled from about four-fifths of an acre to about two-fifths of an acre per head.

Table 5.3), which has increased the amount of family labour available per plot.

Thus, although the intensification of cropping has led to an increased total volume of energy input into agriculture, the concentrated peak jobs, such as ploughing and threshing, have been mechanized, and labour input has only increased in activities such as weeding, which are spread over time and can be handled by the labour of most families. The only manual labour operation for which peak labour is necessary is wheat harvesting, and even with the increased output the village population can handle this by themselves.[11] Through the above mechanisms, labour has been displaced from the village economy in three ways:-

1. Mechanization of male tasks. The operations which have been mechanized are also the only ones which were previously solely the sphere of men, with the result that today most of the labour inputs to agriculture come from women and children.[12] In a significant number of landowning families the men act primarily as managers on their farms, doing this after office hours and at weekends.

2. The employment of wage labourers. It is really only at the wheat harvest time that the landless labourers can be assured of some income from agricultural labour. If combine harvesters were introduced this would also disappear. At other times of the year they may be hired on a casual basis for specific jobs, and wage rates are comparatively high, (Rs. 7-8 per day); but the volume of such employment is not enough to support the entire landless population.

3. Tenancies. The amount of land given out for money, rent or share cropping has declined considerably.[13] Before the advent of mechanization, people used to lease out the land which they could not cultivate with family labour. Now, with the major jobs mechanized, it is possible to cultivate all of one's own land with family labour, supplemented by hired labour if necessary. Thus a major source of subsistence for the smallholders and the landless has been considerably reduced.

---

11. The entire village co-operates to bring in the harvest. People who are employed outside take leave one way or another to do this.
12. Children rarely start work on the land before the age of 11-12, and not in any serious way until they are at least 14 years old.
13. Moreover, a large proportion of the total land leased out seems to go to the wealthy farmers who own tractors. For example, last year a farmer owning 75 bighas and a tractor took in another 80 bighas for sharecropping.

The Impact of Changes in the Village Economy on Different Caste Groups[14]

In the 'traditional' village economy the jajmani system operated, which meant that patron-client relationships existed between individual families of different castes and, more importantly, between the landholding castes and the service castes. The latter were paid in kind by their patrons in exchange for their services. These relationships were hereditary, and therefore secure, although Lewis describes how, even in 1953, they were breaking down. This system has now ceased to exist for most of the service castes, and is dwindling rapidly for the others. In the case of services such as hair-cutting, the breakdown was due to the villagers beginning to obtain these services from the urban sector. For the agricultural labourer caste, the Chamars,[15] the decline in the need for their labour has been described in the previous section. Thus the organic system whereby all castes could derive some living from the land has almost disappeared, and each family has to make its own individual way to secure a living.

Table 5.4 shows the proportion of households in each caste which 'live solely off the land', i.e. directly off the land for the landowners, and indirectly from the provision of services within the village for the rest. The figures give some indication of the volume of labour displaced and the inability of people to live solely off the village economy. Table 5.5 shows for each caste group (1953-1975), the economic opportunities open to them in 1953 and 1975, and the kind of jobs which they held outside the village then and now.

It is not possible to show the same comparisons for the rest of the caste groups in Rampur, since Lewis does not present their population figures separately. However, it can be roughly stated that the position on this table of the higher service castes (carpenter, tailor and barber), would be akin to that of the Brahmins, while that of the lower service castes (potters, washermen) would be closer to that of the sweepers.

Table 5.6 gives a breakdown of the population in each caste group in 1953 and 1975, and their growth rates during this

---

14. This impact is discussed here in terms of caste groups for two reasons. The main one is that occupations (and therefore sources of income) were traditionally defined by caste membership. Changes in the economy tend to affect groups according to the occupation they follow, for example the caste of agricultural labourers were uniformly displaced. The second reason is that the data for 1953 were presented by Lewis in terms of caste rather than class.

15. The Chamars are traditionally not only leatherworkers but also agricultural labourers. This is written into the *wajib-al arz,* the document which specifies the occupations of each caste.

TABLE 5.4

Number of families by caste with no outside income

Caste	Total number of families	Families with no outside source of income	
		Number	Percentage
Jats	143	39	27.2
Brahmins	21	4	19.0
Chamars	30	9	30.0
Bhangis	16	6	37.5
Jhimmers	13	10	76.9
Nai, Bania, Badai, Chippi	19	8	42.1
Lohar, Kumhar Dhobi	13	9	69.2

TABLE 5.5

Caste and changing economic opportunities

Caste	Economic opportunities in the village economy		Types of outside job (predominantly male)	
	1953	1975	1953	1975
1. Jats (land owners)	landowners	land much more productive, but fragmented	white collar, some manual	same as 1953, but greatly expanded
2. Brahmins (priests)	land (small holdings) see Table 5.1	fragmented; less access to modern technology than most Jats, because poorer	white collar	white collar, considerably expanded
	Jajmani: breaking down	broken down		
3. Chamars (agricultural workers)	Jajmani breaking down	broken down, now wage labour; little employment available	some casual labour	some white collar, and some lower income jobs
4. Bhangis (sweepers)	Jajmani sweepers	Jajmani beginning to break down and therefore no longer providing adequate income	some sweeping jobs	mostly sweeping both casual and permanent in nature

TABLE 5.6

Rampur population breakdown and intercensal growth rate by caste

Caste	1953		1975		Intercensal growth rate per annum
	Number	%	Number	%	
Jat (agri-culturists)	648	60.2	1213	60.9	2.9%
Brahmin (priests)	110	10.1	162	8.0	1.76%
Chamar (agricul-tural workers	107	9.9	186	9.2	2.54%
Bhangi (sweepers)	52	4.8	114	5.6	3.63%
Lohar (iron workers)			7		
Jhimmar (water carrier)			83		
Kumhar (potter)			77		
Badai (carpenter)	163	15.0	50	16.3	3.21%
Chippi (tailor)			12		
Dhobi (washerman)			50		
Baniya (shopkeeper)			11		
Nai (barber)			37		
Total	1080	100	2002	100	2.85%

intercensal period.[16] To sum up, -

Caste		Intercensal growth rate per annum
Brahmins	- already in urban jobs to a large extent by 1953	1.75%
Chamars	- beginning to move into urban jobs in 1960's	2.54%
Bhangis	- still half inside the village economy	3.63%

It is apparent from the data that the Brahmins, who have been operating longest in the urban economy, had a significantly slower growth rate than the rest of the village population.[17] Those who have continued to operate within the village economy, or on casual labour (the sweepers), have been growing fastest at a rate which is high by any standards. The Chamars may have started to limit their fertility, but as yet it is hard to tell because they have been phased out of the village economy fairly recently.

The Jats are far less homogeneous than other castes since they are the landowners, and there is a great deal of variation in their income levels according to size of landholding and participation in the wider economy. With regard to their fertility behaviour, it is only possible to say that the fact of owning land whose high productivity has so far been constantly increasing presumably makes the perceived need for small families less pressing for all but the poorest. Nowadays, for the majority of the Jats, fragmentation of holdings, mechanization, and the ever-growing desire to obtain white-collar urban jobs, might make for their wanting to limit their family size. In fact only the richest can meet all the necessary expenses for several children.[18]

---

16. These intercensal growth rates (natural rate of increase per annum) have been computed from the total population in each caste as enumerated in 1953 and 1975. Data collected on migration shows that net migration has had a negligible effect on these population totals.
17. Since it was not the traditional occupation of the higher service castes to operate other people's land, they were the first to respond to the breakdown of the organic village economy by taking advantage of opportunities external to the village.
18. It is more difficult nowadays to solve the problem of small-holdings by taking in land for sharecropping. Also, very little of the village land ever comes onto the market, because most people supplement their income from outside sources - thereby avoiding the vicious circle of land sale and debt well known in India.

TABLE 5.7

Approximate annual costs of educating a child, 1975

Type of expense	Primary Education (Rs.)	Higher Secondary (Rs.)	Higher education (Rs.)	
			Living at home	Living in hostel
Fees	15[a]	80[b]	300	3,000 including board
Books etc.	25	50	100	200
Travel	-	-	70	200
Clothes	50	65[c]	250	500[d]
Pocket expenses	25	50	110[e]	500
Total	115	245	830	4,400

a) Fees range from Rs. 12 - 20.

b) Fees range from Rs. 60 -100.

c) Clothes expenditure ranges from Rs. 60 - 70.

d) Clothes expenditure ranges from Rs. 400 -600.

e) Pocket expenses range from Rs. 80 - 150.

TABLE 5.8

Approximate salaries for different urban jobs and corresponding educational levels required, 1975

Jobs	Approx. monthly salaries (Rs.)	Educational requirements
Army/Police	600+	Higher Secondary (H.S.)
Teacher	800 - 1,000	B.A. + Teacher's Training
White collar	400 - 600	B.A.
Transport	400 - 600	H.S. / B.A.
Factory work	300 - 600	H.S. / B.A.
Low permanent	200	H.S.

The Implications for Fertility

Fertility decline is not brought about merely by increased integration in the industrial-urban economy. People's fertility behaviour is crucially affected by the *kinds* of jobs in the urban economy to which they aspire and stand a chance of getting. Two types of jobs are available: either casual jobs, or permanent salaried jobs. The latter offer a steady source of income and sometimes in addition a pension, which is very important for old age security.[19] It is clear, both from what people say and from how they allocate their money, that the villagers want permanent jobs for themselves and their children.

These secure jobs are the ones for which heavy investments in terms of time and money are necessary. Table 5.7 gives an indication of the costs involved in educating a child, and Table 5.8 shows the advertised levels required for different urban jobs and the wages associated with them. Bribes for clerical and army jobs are of the order of Rs. 1,000-2,000 and it is often necessary to pay this bribe several times before getting a job because the bribe-taker does not fulfil his promises. This extra element of risk makes the poorer people even less likely to get jobs, because they are averse to spending all their savings on a one-time risk. If they lose the bribe, they have no savings left, either to live on or to use for the next bribe.

The higher castes had a monopoly of the better jobs in 1953 (see Table 5.2) and, with the exception of the Jats, were highly dependent on these for their income. By 1975, the agricultural labourer caste (Chamar) had started moving into these jobs (see Table 5.9) and the degree of dependence of all castes on the outside economy had increased considerably. The service castes which are still half within the village economy (i.e. sweepers) tend to remain confined to sweeping jobs, often casual in nature, in the outside economy.[20]

Each caste group is acquiring education to a level corresponding with their employment situations (see Table 5.10). Table 5.11 shows the great increase in the volume of education since 1953. By 1975 the lower service castes had started acquiring education to a considerable extent. They are trying to move into the better jobs, but are hindered by their difficulties in raising the bribe-component of the necessary investment.

---

19. A pension relieves the concern for old-age security, which is often stated as a reason for wanting children.
20. The Chamars as a group have succeeded better than the sweepers in exploiting the new opportunities presented by the Government's pro-untouchable caste policies, partly because they are a bigger group, and have more contacts to manipulate in the urban sphere.

TABLE 5.9

Distribution of urban occupations by caste, 1975

Caste	Total no. of men age 15-64 in each caste group	Percent employed in urban economy	Percentage distribution of urban employed in different sectors							
			Army/ Police	Teachers	White* Collar	Transport	Factory Workers	Self** Employed	Low+ Permanent	Sweepers
Jats	354	42.6	16.5	20.61	22.61	14.6	13.2	1.3	11.2	0
Brahmins	55	61.8	5.8	29.4	41.21	2.9	17.6	0	2.9	0
Chamars	50	50.0	12.0	0	32.0	0	20.0	8.0	28.0	0
Bhangis	22	63.6	0	0	0	0	21.4	0	14.2	64.41
Jhimmers	20	15.0	0	0	0	0	0	0	100.0	0
Nai, Banai, Badai, Chippi	32	59.3	21.21	47.51	5.2	5.2	10.5	5.2	5.2	0
Lohar, Kumhar, Dhobi	43	18.6	25.0	0	0	0	12.5	12.5	50.0	0

* Clerks, Post Office, etc.

** Trading and selling milk and vegetables etc.

\+ Peons etc.

TABLE 5.10

Education by caste, 1975

Highest educational level attained / Caste	Jat	Brahmin	Chamar	Bhangi	Jhimmer	Nai, Bania, Badai, Chippi	Lohar, Kumhar, Dhobi
(Total population in caste-group	1213	162	186	114	83	110	95
1 - 4 years	176	27	37	14	9	18	22
5 - 8 years	223	26	35	9	8	30	20
9 - Higher secondary	277	42	26	1	2	20	18
BA +	25	10	0	0	0	6	1
Teacher's training	33	4	1	0	0	6	0
Total	734	109	99	24	19	80	61
% Educated	60.5	67.2	53.2	21.0	22.8	72.7	64.2

TABLE 5.11

School attendance by caste, 1953

		Jat	Brahmin	Chamar	Bhangi	Jhimmer	Nai, Bania, Badai, Chippi	Lomar, Kumhar, Dhobi
Percent Males (age 6-15)	M	92	84	86	0	67	100	20
Percent Females (age 6-15)	F	40	30	6	0	0	50	0

This discrepancy between educational level and job attainment applies also, though to a lesser extent, to the Chamars.

These changes in access to education and economic opportunities have brought about a fairly sharp division of the population into two groups, each of which is differentially placed in terms of exploiting these opportunities. It can be seen further that membership of one group or another has important implications for fertility behaviour.

The first group consists of those who have some surplus, either from agricultural or non-agricultural income. This capital is the *sine qua non* of success. It is only through the accumulation of a certain amount of wealth that an individual can firstly have access to education, and secondly obtain the much-prized urban job by paying the necessary bribe. Once having acquired some education and being in a better position to perceive ways of exploiting his new opportunities, it is likely that there will be a significant change in his fertility behaviour. In order to continue his own upward spiral, and also to pass on to his children the benefits which the new opportunities present, one may expect that he will adopt the norm of the small family. The motivation is present and the means are available.

The second group, on the other hand, finds it more difficult to improve its present position. Since the initial investment necessary to procure education and urban employment is lacking, members of this group never reach the take-off point which will enable them to exploit the new opportunities. They are victims of the 'paradox of poverty', in which the nature of the economic opportunities (casual jobs and their traditional services) open to them dictates that the optimal course of action is for them to have large numbers of children, and thereby maximize the expected current income for the family. At any rate, this may be their thinking before the event, but later some families may find that this does not succeed. Moreover, it exacerbates the problem of reaching the necessary take-off point into the upward spiral.[21]

This indicates that it is not an extreme level of poverty (stemming from losing a foothold in the village economy) which makes for fertility decline, but rather that a minimal degree of affluence is necessary to motivate people to control the number of their children so as to best exploit the new opportunities.

---

21. One possible course of action for these people would be to invest all the resources acquired from the earnings of large numbers of children, towards enabling one of their children to 'take off' into a good job. However, judging by the results, they do not seem to be succeeding in this, even if they are trying to do so.

The Effect of Education and Employment on Age at Marriage and Attitudes to Family Size

The average age at marriage in Rampur is rising, at least partly through the effects of education and employment. Education directly affects age at marriage, because girls and boys tend to wait until they have finished their education before marrying, or at least before beginning to cohabit permanently. Moreover, for the upper strata education is becoming increasingly a qualification for marriage. Both education and employment tend to raise age at marriage and reduce desired family size, thereby in two ways contributing to a slower growth rate. The following are some of the mechanisms whereby the attitudes are changed:-

1. Contact with urban norms (little of this happens in the context of village schools, so it really takes place with higher education).

2. Educated, employed parents want their children to follow in their footsteps, and the expenses involved put a premium on lower fertility.

3. Employed women have less time to look after their children.

4. Educated, employed parents may have better knowledge of the contraceptive methods available, how to gain access to them, and be able to use them effectively.

Whereas most of the older women in the village think of five children as a good number to have, there are many highly-educated young women (a few of whom are employed as school-teachers) who think in terms of having three children and then being sterilized. Although these women are aware of the advantages of birth-spacing, the strength of the norms of their parental generation make it important for them to have their desired number of children first, before using any contraception.

Of the village data collected, a 100% KAP study and extensive maternity histories of a stratified sample still remain to be analysed. However, it can be stated that conversations with the villagers and with the local doctor suggested that couples belonging to a variety of castes and income groups are practising contraception, but mostly favour terminal methods.

The Government Family Planning Programme

In view of the fact that there is a considerable volume of felt need for contraception in the village, it is interesting to see how far the Government family planning programme manages to meet these needs. The programme has been integrated with the provision of general health facilities for rural areas, all of which is carried out from Primary Health Centres (PHC's). Each of these centres caters for several villages. The PHC serving

Plate I

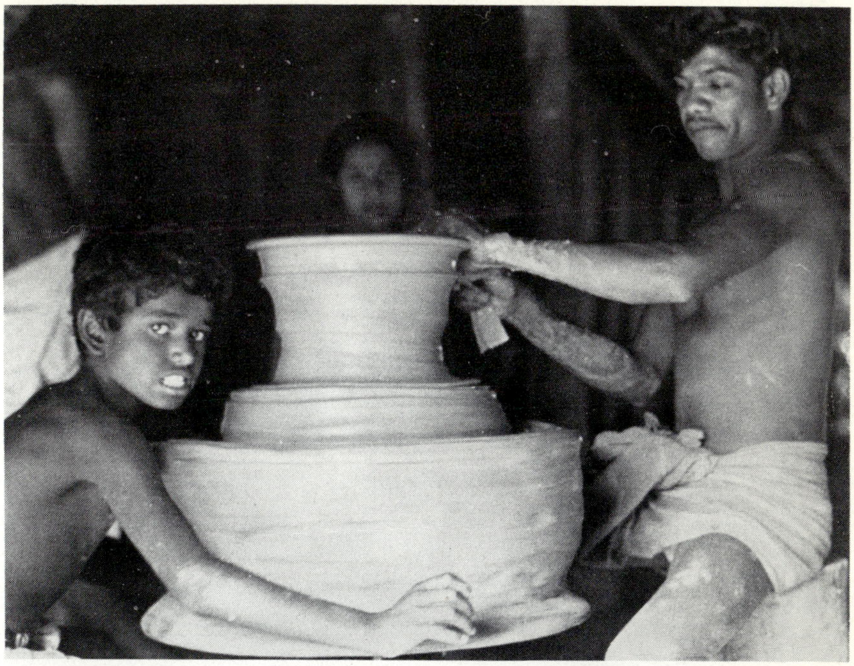

Village potter in Aluthgama-Bogamuwa
(Photo: W. M. Tilakaratne)

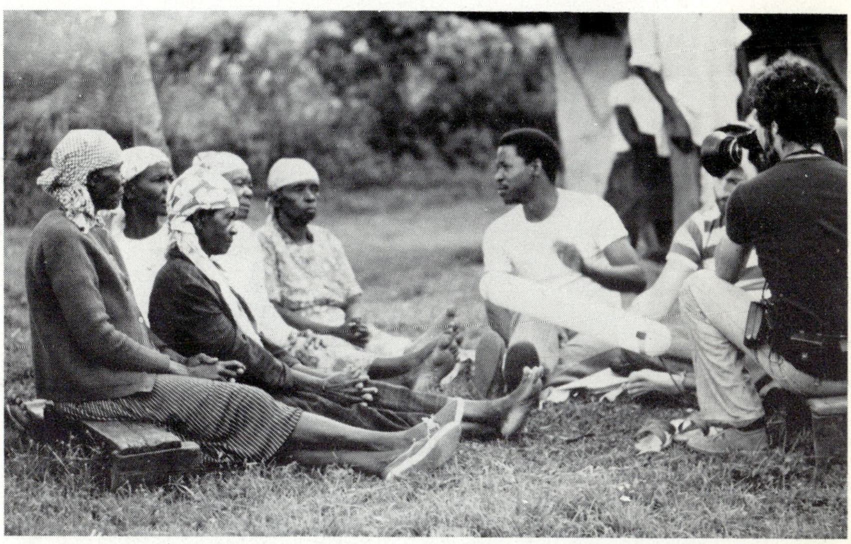

Joseph Ssenyonga discusses fertility during filming in Maragoli (Photo: Sandra Nichols)

Plate II

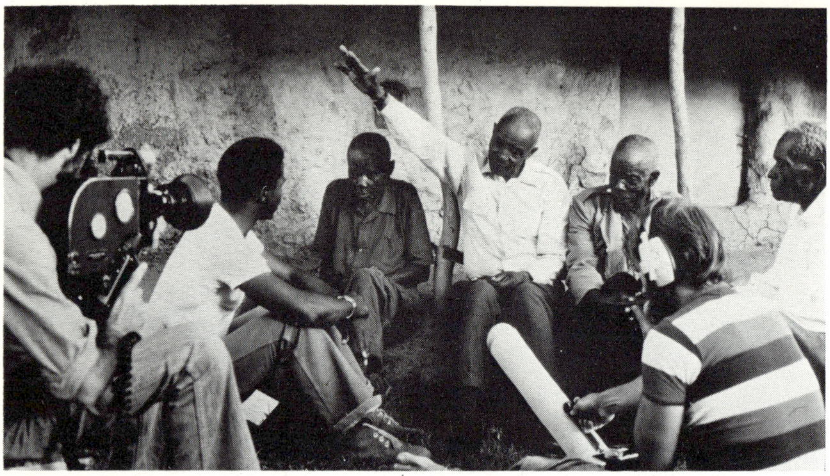

A village elder makes a point during filming
(Photo: Sandra Nichols)

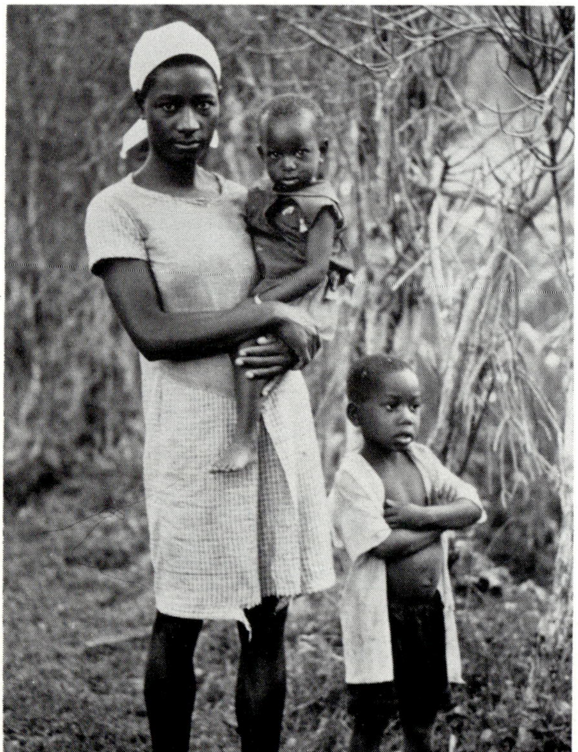

Mother and children in Maragoli
(Photo: Sandra Nichols)

Plate III

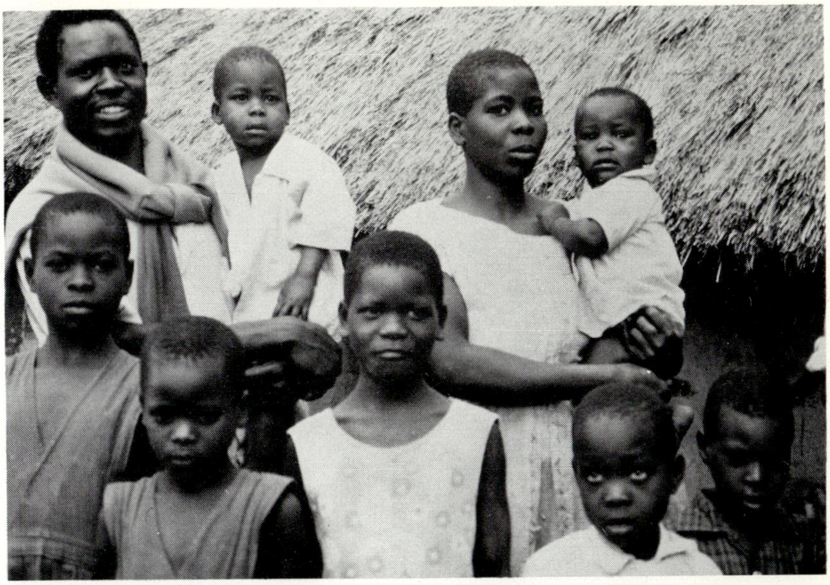

Maragoli family (Photo: Sandra Nichols)

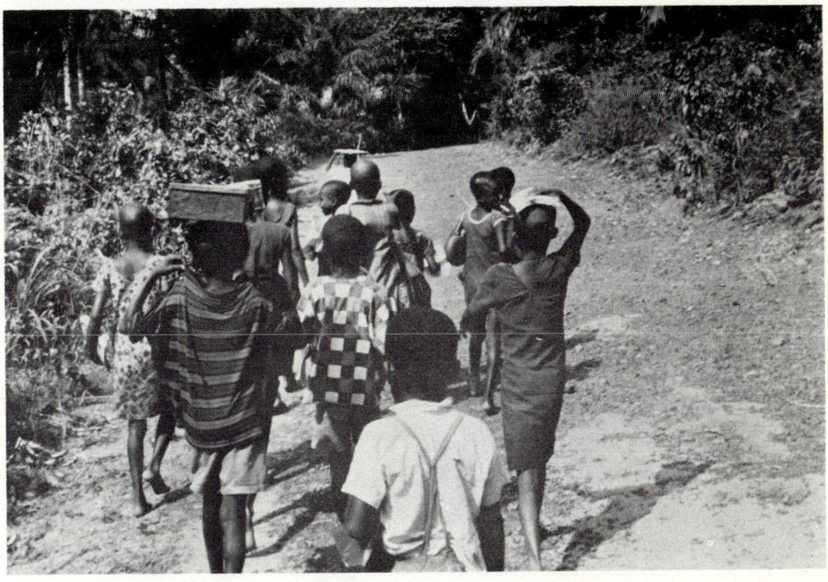

The burden of knowledge: daily journey to school in Umueke (Photo: Sandra Nichols)

Plate IV

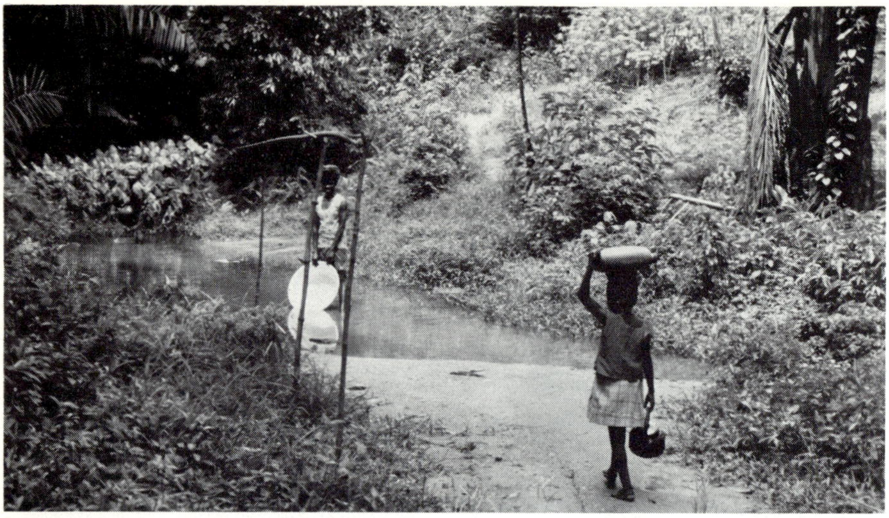

Fetching water from the village pond (Photo: Sandra Nichols)

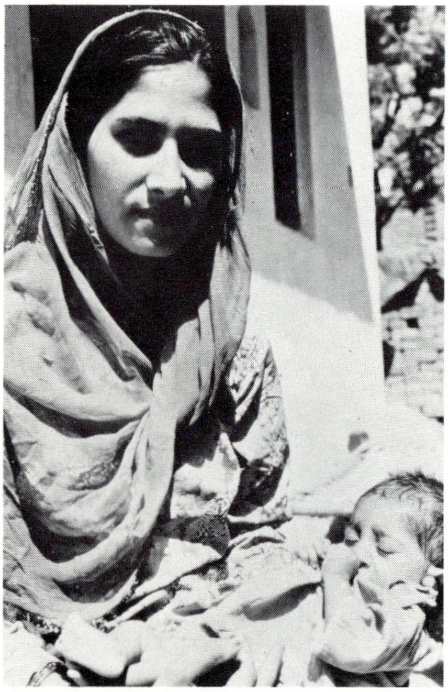

Jat mother and child, Rampur (Photo: Sandra Nichols)

Plate V

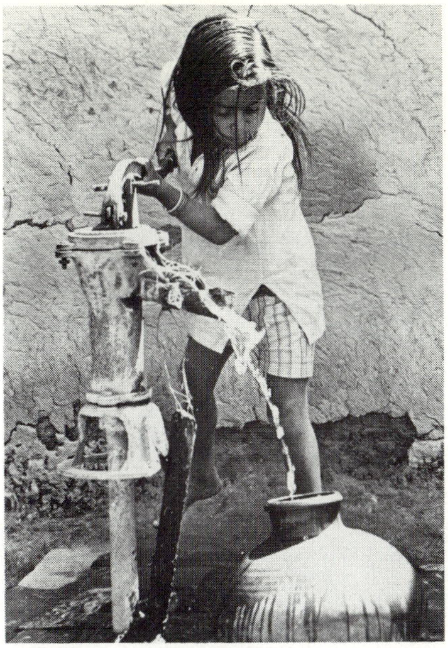

One of several daily visits to the well
(Photo: Sandra Nichols)

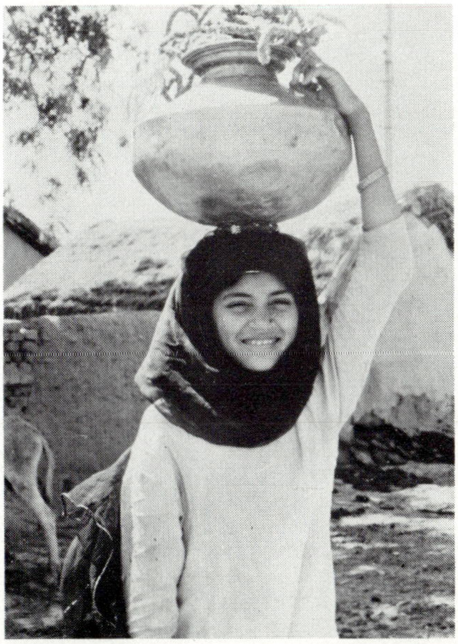

Children contribute labour to the family at an early age
(Photo: Mukul Dube)

Plate VI

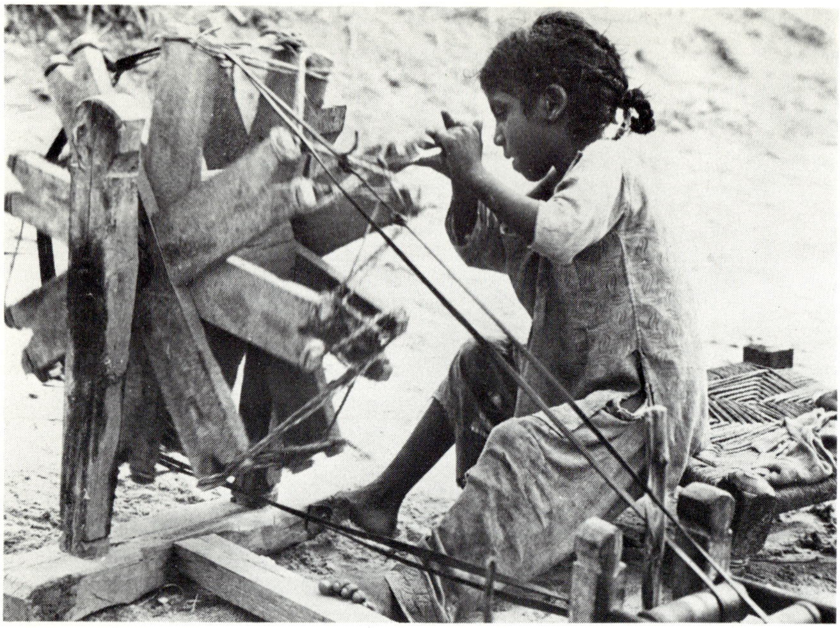

Rope making in Mulkipure (Photo: Mukul Dube)

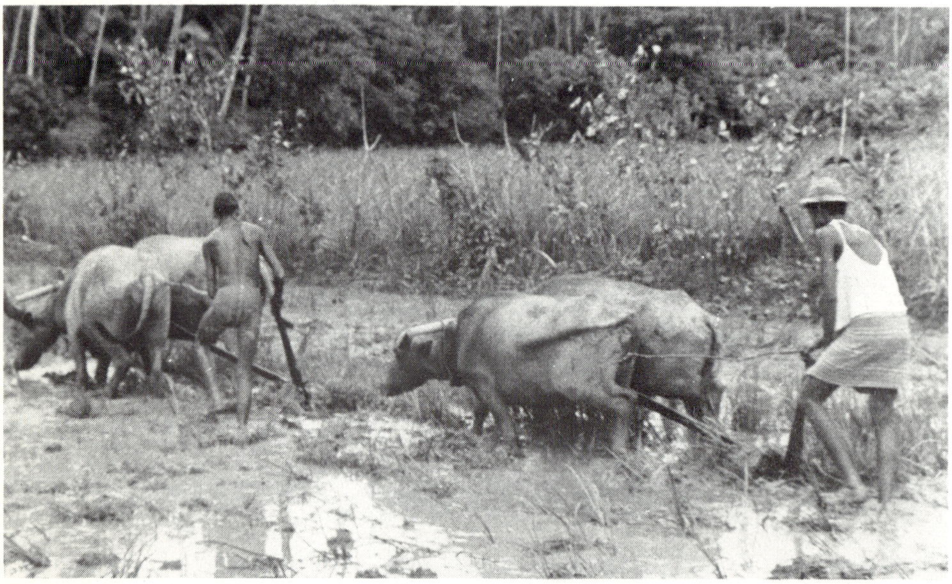

Ploughing paddy land in Delumgoda (Photo: W. M. Tilakaratne)

Plate VII

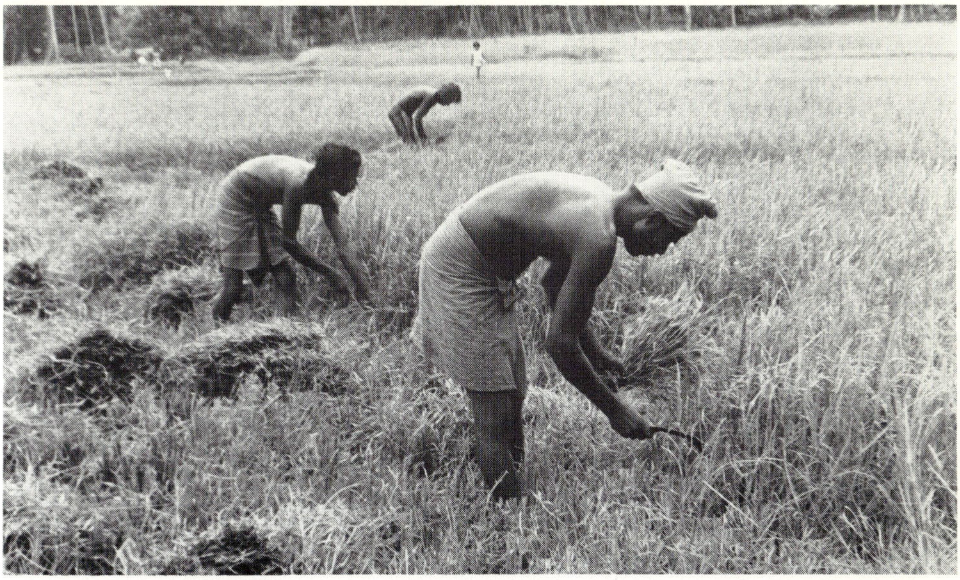

Cutting fodder in Delumgoda (Photo: W. M. Tilakaratne)

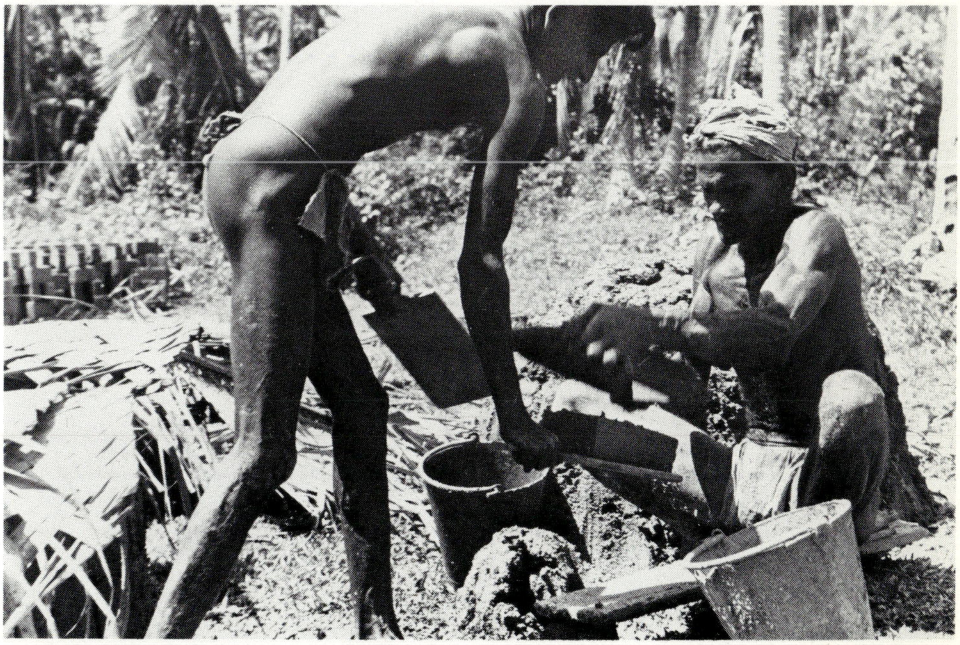

Brickmaking in Aluthgama-Bogamuwa (Photo: W. M. Tilakaratne)

Plate VIII

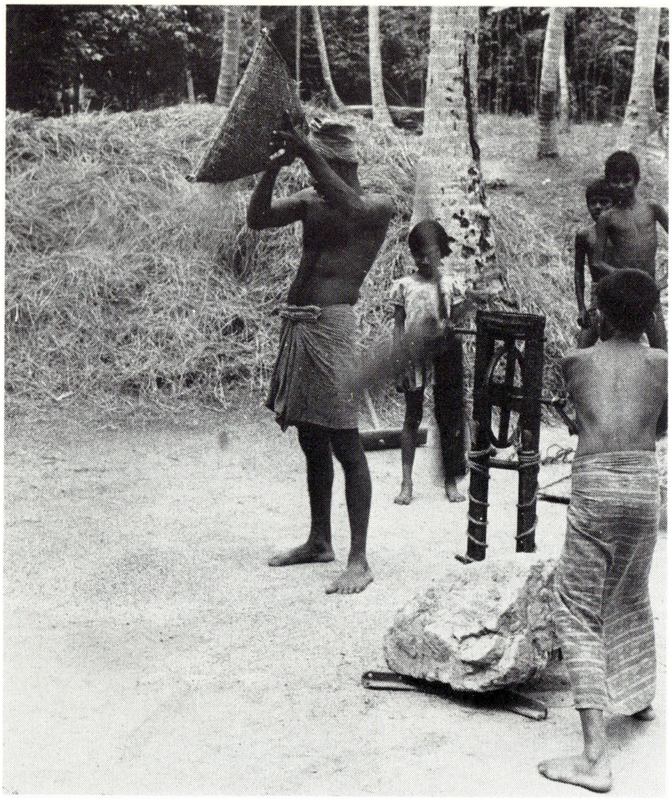

Winnowing with hand-operated fan
(Photo: W. M. Tilakaratne)

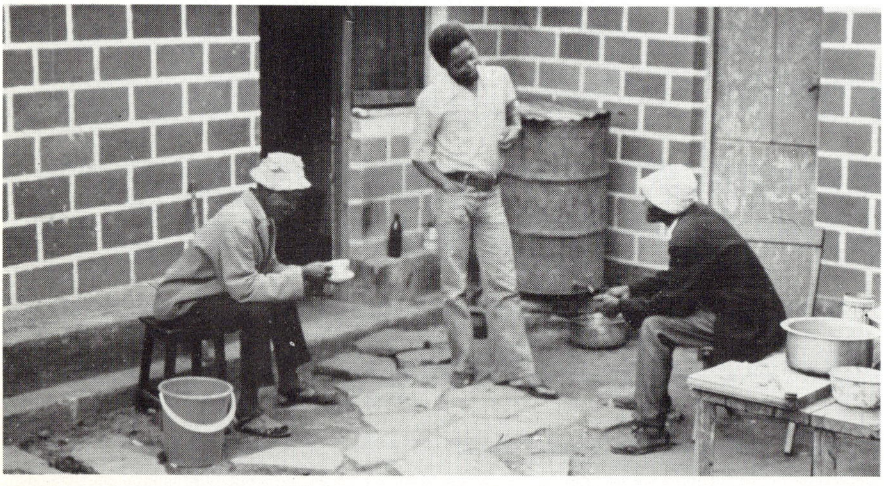

Author with villagers in Taita-Taveta (Photo: Sandra Nichols)

Plate IX

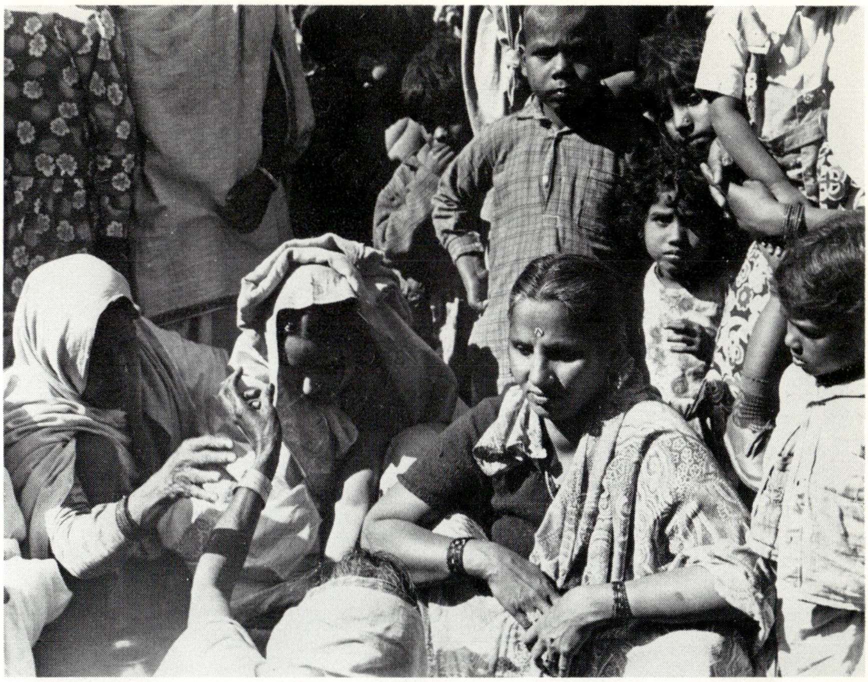

Thakur bride-to-be is blessed in the Dhobi quarter of Ramaua (Photo: Mukul Dube)

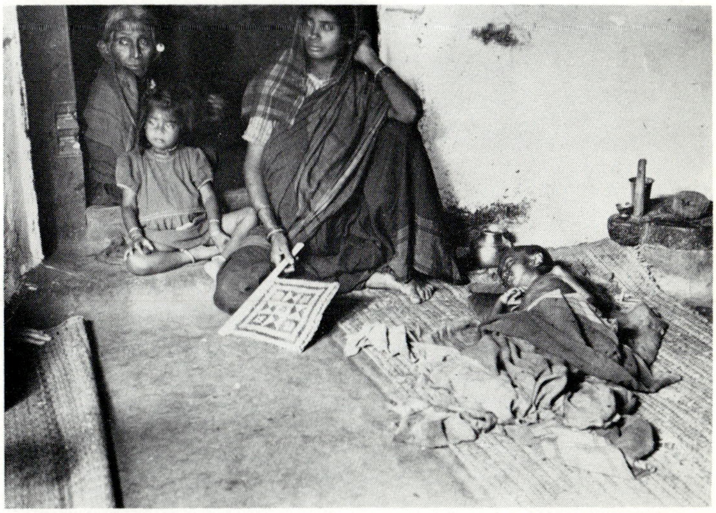

A mother mourns the death of her child in an Indian villate (Photo: Scarlett Epstein)

Plate X

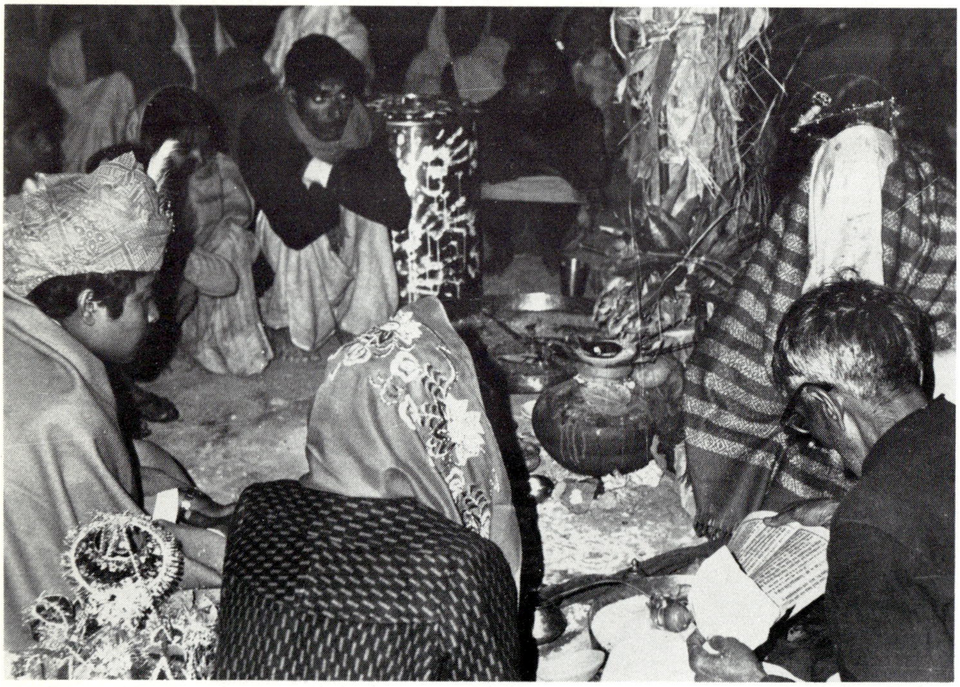

Ramaua marriage: groom, bride and priest (Photo: Mukul Dube)

Rampur is just over a mile away from the village, and services a total population of 60,000. When fully staffed, there are two doctors, one gynaecologist-cum-family planning organizer, and a large body of healthworkers (field staff) for family planning, malaria, and smallpox, which includes trained midwives. Being so close to Delhi, this PHC is better staffed, funded and run than most in rural India. The present team of doctors is highly qualified and dedicated, but it cannot cope with the volume of patients. Also, the PHC is always short of drugs. On the other hand the large body of assorted health workers do very little, but absorb a good deal of the resources allocated to the health services, in terms of salaries.[22] The monthly expenditure on staff salaries in this PHC is Rs. 19,000.

The villagers of Rampur tend to believe in things which they have seen will work. They are not guided solely by their traditional belief systems. For example, they adopted the new agricultural technology very quickly (similarly with smallpox vaccinations), because they see that it works. But in the face of drug shortages the doctors cannot always help their patients. Thus the villagers see the doctors - and consequently their medical system - as fallible.

It is very important to increase people's faith in the contraceptive and general medical technology being offered them. This can be best done by closely linking-up the family planning services with general maternal and child care services. Such integration exists in the conceptualisation of the family planning programme at the planning level, but little of it is reflected in practice. Even basic jobs, such as after-care of women who have been sterilized or have had IUDs inserted are not adequately done. As for the trained midwives, they attend only a fraction of the births in the villages,nor do they give much care before or after a birth. They are not usually available at night, when a lot of births take place. The villagers feel that the midwife will come to them only if they can make her some gift - it should be added that the midwifery services are supposed to be free. Consequently most childbirths are handled by the villagers themselves with the help of the traditional village midwife, although the villagers feel that the trained midwife is more skilled. Most of the abortions are also handled by the villagers themselves or by quacks. The health services ought to be able to cater for the demand for abortions, if only because do-it-yourself abortions are extremely dangerous for the mother's health.

Lack of proper communication has meant that there is a fair amount of unmet felt need for contraception. For example, one women who was having her ninth child was complaining about

---

22. Another example of wastage of resources is the distribution of free condoms. The doctor has to persuade the workers to distribute them, and they tend to end up being given to people who would probably have bought them in the market.

endless childbearing, and when I asked her why she did not have herself sterilized, she said that she was uncertain about what this would involve. This unmet felt need could be far better satisfied if efforts were made to explain the various methods of contraception to the villagers, and to gear these methods to meet their individual needs.[23] As it is, the villagers believe that there are only three methods of contraception available - sterilization, IUD and condoms. In spite of the family planning services they have very little knowledge of other methods, such as the pill.

There is a tremendous urban bias in the organization and staffing of the PHCs. The clinic workers feel that they are superior to the patients from the villages, and this feeling of superiority reflects itself in their behaviour. They treat the villagers as inferior beings, and as an undifferentiated mass of people who need to be harangued to do anything rational, whereas what the patients need is a recognition of their individual needs, and an attempt to help them fulfill them. Thus the doctors and the gynaecologist sit in their rooms, swamped by a stream of patients. All the doctors can do, as far as family planning propagation is concerned, is to catch some of the women as they come to the clinic, and try to persuade them to adopt family planning. They don't have the time to sit and explain the mechanics of different methods and persuade them to adopt one or other method. Faced by a team of people (doctor and lower-level workers) who are constantly hectoring them, the villagers become defensive in their attitude, feeling that their own values and needs are not understood by these people, that the gap is unbridgeable - that somehow, if they can only get their medicine and escape, they will be happy. This is not a conducive atmosphere for propagating family planning.

Thus, in the village, the Government family planning programme does not succeed even in meeting the total felt need for contraception. Not only should this existing need be met, but it should be increased. For instance, the villagers should be encouraged to use spacing methods more than they do. At present they are becoming aware of the advantages of birth spacing, but still use terminal methods (male and female sterilization, and IUD used as a terminal method).

Altogether, the PHC, although it is relatively well-run and many resources are spent on it, caters for a small fraction of the total demand for medical services and a somewhat bigger fraction of the total demand for family planning in the village.

The villagers meet another fraction of their needs by going to other rural doctors (belonging to other systems of medicine) or to quacks, or to Delhi. Even in a village which has access to medical services in Delhi a good deal of the total felt need for health and family planning services remains unmet.

---

23. Contraceptive technology is also clearly a problem, and needs to be improved.

Conclusion

In this paper I examined the relationship between the very significant differences in the growth rate of different sections of Rampur on the one hand, and the different economic opportunities open to these villagers, on the other. The Brahmins, who have for the longest period been dependent on the urban economy for much of their income, have had a considerably lower growth rate than those who remained in the village economy. With the growth of population and the mechanization of agriculture, an increasing proportion of villagers is seeking urban employment.

However, the various rural strata are differentially equipped to avail themselves of the external employment opportunities, which is reflected in the rationale of their fertility behaviour. The upper strata find it easier to secure the better paid permanent jobs, simply because they are in a position to meet the heavy but necessary investment in education and bribes. The volume of investment thus required puts a premium on lower fertility and helps to explain the increasing interest among this group to limit their family size.

Of the lower strata, only some have struggled to make these investments and thereby managed to get a foothold on the upward spiral to economic success. However, the bulk of the poorer strata cannot afford such heavy expenditure and have to rely on their traditional village occupations and casual jobs for their subsistence. These people hope to maximize their potential income by having large numbers of children, which in turn makes it increasingly difficult for them to get onto the upward spiral.

The existing Government Family Planning services are inadequate to meet even the presently felt need for contraception in Rampur, far from expanding it or encouraging couples to space their children.

I have attempted to delineate the actual mechanisms through which education and industrialization are influencing fertility in Rampur. The changes which have occurred in the wider socio-economic environment have been mediated by group norms. For this reason it may be expected that fertility decline is not confined solely to those people who have benefitted most from the new economic opportunities. It can be assumed that other factors influencing fertility behaviour (e.g. religious beliefs) apply equally to all groups, thus there is reason to believe that changing fertility behaviour is a response to a changing economic environment. Attempts to explain such changes must take into account the nature of the different options open to different groups within a society undergoing a transition from a peasant to an industrialized society.

APPENDIX 5.1

Rampur demographic indices

The average annual growth rate over the period 1953-1975 is 2.85% p.a.

The Total Fertility Rate = 7.5

The growth rate is very high, and this, along with the shape of the age pyramid (Chart 5.1), suggests that while fertility is very high, mortality has been declining for some time now.

This overall picture is supported by the figures for Haryana State. These figures also throw light on the possible demographic developments over time in the Rampur area.

% Decadal growth, 1901-71, Haryana State

	% growth over decade	
1901 - 1911	- 9.70	period during which Darling (1947) states that heavy emigration was taking place to the newly irrigated areas further west, and population was growing slower than the land under cultivation.
1911 - 1921	+ 1.95	
1921 - 1931	+ 7.14	
1931 - 1941	+ 15.63	
1941 - 1951	+ 7.60	
1951 - 1961	+ 33.79	
1961 - 1971	+ 31.36	

The data indicates possible heavy emigration in the first decade or two. Thereafter the population started growing steadily. The rate of growth increases in a way which suggests the beginning of steady mortality decline at least by the 1930's. The 1941-51 figures are complicated by the fact of the mass migrations which took place in 1948-1950 during the partition of India and Pakistan.

In either the 1940's or the 1950's, mortality must have declined heavily, because the rate of growth becomes very high. This is the period of most rapid population growth. The figure for 1961-71 shows that the population is still growing very fast, but growth appears to have slowed down.

Haryana is one of the only four Indian states (out of a total of eighteen) which shows this slowing down of growth. Fertility is still very high (as it is in Rampur), but is showing signs of decreasing. This could be the beginnings of the third stage of the demographic transition.

CHART 5.1

Rampur 1953 and 1974: age/sex pyramid

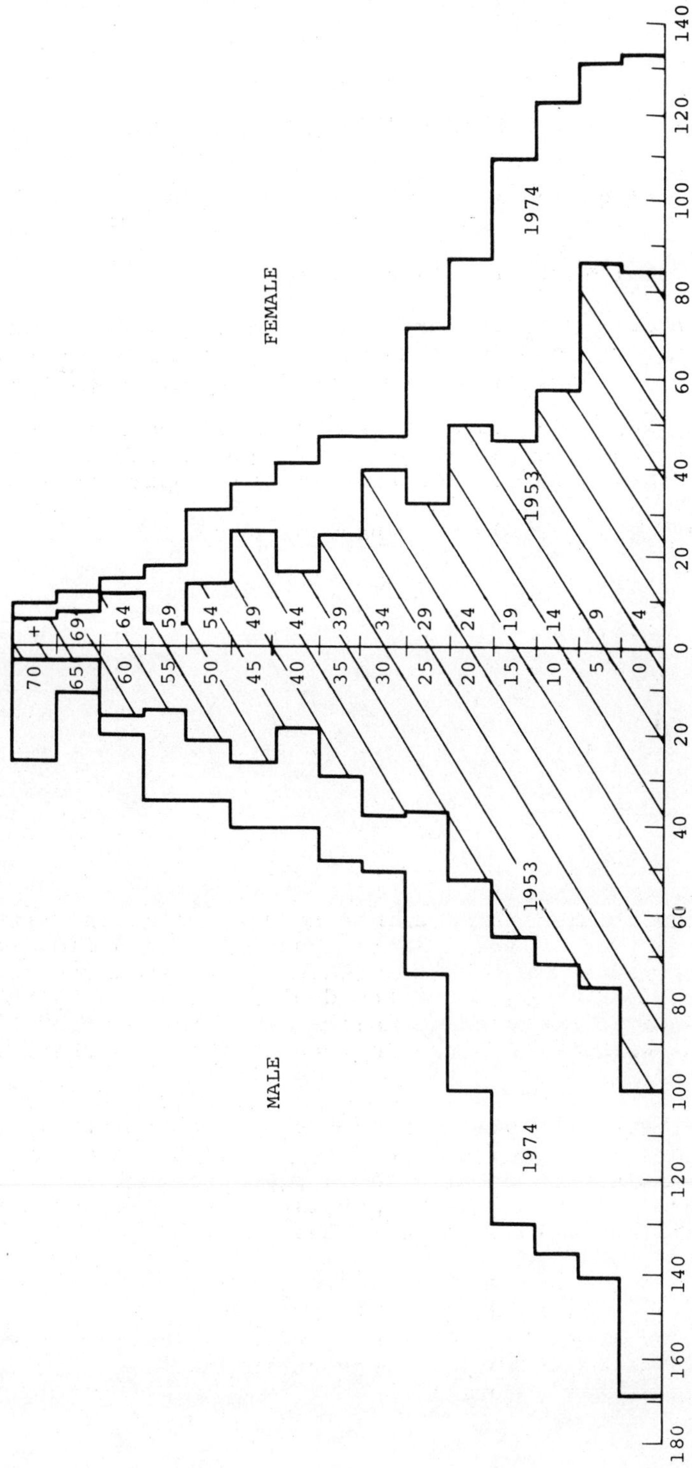

PART 3

DEVELOPMENT AND FERTILITY

CHAPTER 6

INTRA-RURAL MIGRATION IN A NORTH INDIAN DISTRICT

Studies of migration have so far concerned themselves principally with the following phenomena: urbanisation; movement of workers to semi-urban places of employment; movement of people between administrative entities, within a country or internationally; and the cultural adaptation of immigrants. The reasons for such limitations of interest are not difficult to identify. Each of these phenomena has been of considerable importance in a number of places at various times: urbanisation has universally accompanied the commercial and industrial development of societies and has been a by-product of overloading in rural sectors; the labour forces of many semi-urban productive ventures - some properly industrial, some less so, e.g. mines - have had to be drawn from other regions; large-scale shifts of population between administrative units have always been a source of concern to the administrations involved; and problems have often arisen in the course of the cultural assimilation of immigrant groups.

Additionally, demographers and other social scientists interested in the study of migration have had to rely almost entirely on data already collected and available. These data have tended to relate to the phenomena mentioned above because of two features which are common to them. In all cases migration is either permanent or for substantial periods of time; and in all cases large numbers of people are involved. Each of these factors is critical - and their combination even more so - for the convenient availability of reliable data and, indeed, for the very need to gather such data for purposes of administration and management.

Thus short-term migration, even if large numbers of people are involved and even if such migration occurs frequently or in a regular cycle, has tended to be ignored. A.P. Katti, for instance, who found 170 outside labourers spending over 20 weeks each working in a village in Mysore state (now Karnataka), dismissed the matter as unimportant because the immigrant casual labourers amounted to only 4% of the village population (Katti, 1966).

In regions in India where substantial localised progress in agriculture has been achieved there is a great need for labour to handle seasonally determined agricultural tasks. Locally available labour is often not sufficient to cope, hence labour has to be drawn from other regions to meet these specific needs. Such temporarily migrating casual labourers perform an essential function and as such are vital to the agricultural economy of the region in which they undertake seasonal work.

In addition to regional imbalance in agricultural potential and development there are in India numerous instances of imbalance in commercial and industrial development; the two kinds of imbalance often occur together. The implications of this for the employment potential and employment structure of regions are obvious. Some regions are rendered more able than others to absorb labour either in the agrarian sector or in the urban-industrial sector or in both. Thus situations of labour shortage and labour surplus are created.

Demographic factors are naturally of immense importance. Population pressure is experienced when a region either cannot produce enough of the items necessary to the existence of its population, or is unable to provide sufficiently paying employment for its working population. These two conditions often occur together. For a variety of reasons there are inter-regional differences both in terms of absolute population size and in terms of ability to cope with populations by the two means noted above.

To summarise then, differences in agricultural and industrial development combine with differences in population size and structure to produce significant regional imbalances in terms of the availability of employment and the nature of employment available. The ultimate expression of population pressure in a region of low overall development is invariably surplus labour. The only course open in such a situation - in the absence of devices such as social security programmes and massive investment from sources external to the region - is migration in search of work.

The place to which migration occurs and its duration are determined largely by the nature of the work available and also by the abilities of the workers migrating. Whatever the specific features of a case, however, the formation of a labour market more extensive than previously existing ones is an important development. In any system of production - especially those of semi-industrial societies - labour is in purely economic terms an important means of production. In addition to this, and perhaps more significantly, labour is the only *human* means of production in a human society. Finally, as discussed earlier, questions that are of paramount concern to developing nations (overpopulation in relation to resource availability) find expression ultimately in the problems of labour.

In broad terms this forms the justification for any study of labour. More pointedly it forms the justification for studying temporary (seasonally repetitive) migration of agricultural labourers to regions which could not manage without this additional input. This kind of migration is the basis of the present paper.

Mulkipur, the village to which the migrant group studied belongs, is situated in the northern part of Saharanpur district in western Uttar Pradesh (UP). Broadly speaking, agricultural production and the general standard of living show gradual improvement as one moves from eastern to western UP, and more improvement further west in Haryana and Punjab states. Western UP, Haryana and Punjab are India's major producers of wheat and sugarcane and north India's largest producers of rice. Seen in comparison with the rest of India, western UP is an agriculturally productive region. Also it does not exhibit the extremes of poverty that other parts of India do. This should not, however, be taken to mean that the region is actually a prosperous one.

Saharanpur district, roughly put, falls outside the north-eastern boundary of the industrialising belt stretching north-west from Delhi. It has few industries except for a prestige public sector corporation manufacturing electrical goods and a factory of the India (formerly Imperial) Tobacco Company. The district has had, for over a century, large numbers of wood-carvers and metalworkers but these occupations are now suffering from a glut of labour and a shortage of markets. The other minor industries in the region - sugar mills, units manufacturing cardboard, etc. - are in a relatively frozen state; they are not growing and are in no position to absorb more labour. In sum, the urban-industrial employment available, either to urban workers or to displaced agricultural labourers, is minimal throughout the district.

There is some variation through the district in terms of agricultural development. The southern portion bordering Muzaffarnagar district and the western portion bordering Haryana state are relatively well developed in that productivity is high and modern techniques, seeds, etc., are being used. Arguably one of the important reasons for the greater prosperity of these parts of the district is the availability of water from the Eastern Yamuna Canal. Mulkipur falls in that part of the district which does not have access to this water and moreover has a rather sandy and infertile kind of soil. In short, Mulkipur shares with the rest of the district a lack of industrial employment, being a little worse off, in fact, because it is at the northern end and thus physically farther away. Agriculturally, it is distinctly behind in terms of productivity and effective use of modern technology.

I shall now describe briefly the position of the migrant workers in Mulkipur and the various forces that have caused them to seek agricultural work outside their own village.

Mulkipur is a large village of both Hindu and Muslim castes. The caste distribution is given in Table 6.1. It will be seen that the principal landholding caste are the Siyanis. Some households of the Badhi and Vaish castes also own substantial holdings. Among the Muslim castes only some Gada households have large holdings.

The distribution of landholdings, caste-wise, is given in Table 6.2, which shows that a large part of Mulkipur's population is made up of landless households and those with extremely small holdings. (Incidentally, there is a reference in the

TABLE 6.1

Caste composition of Mulkipur

Hindu castes	No. of households
Siyani (agriculturist)	70
Brahman (priest)	1
Vaish (merchant)	4
Dhiman (carpenter)	7
Kumhar (potter)	1
Bairagi (priest)	1
Kahar (oven-owner)	3
Balar (scavenger)	14
Chamar (leatherworker)	70
Muslim castes	
Teli (oil-presser)	33
Gada (agriculturist)	11
Fakir (mendicant)	6
Nai (barber)	4
Sakka (water-carrier)	2
Dhobi (washerman)	1
Total	228

TABLE 6.2

Land distribution in Mulkipur by caste

bighas*	Bairagi	Balar	Brahman	Chamar	Dhiman	Dhobi	Fakir	Gada	Kahar	Kumhar	Nai	Sakka	Siyani	Teli	Vaish	Total
LANDLESS	1	14		47	2	1	6	1		1	4	2	6	23		108
0 - 10				12	2				3				4	2		23
10 - 20				8	1			2					11	2	1	25
20 - 30				2									9	2		13
30 - 40			1	1				4					11	1	1	19
40 - 50					1			1					7	2	1	12
50 - 60					1								8	1		10
60 - 70													4			4
70 - 80													1			1
80 - 90								1					3		1	5
90 -100								1					2			3
100 -110													1			1
125								1								1
180													1			1
190													1			1
200													1			1
Total	1	14	1	70	7	1	6	11	3	1	4	2	70	33	4	228

* 5 bighas = 1 acre (approx.)

TABLE 6.3

Population distribution by sex and caste and average household size in Mulkipur

	MALE	FEMALE	TOTAL
Chamars	169	143	312
Balars	30	32	62
All others	652	550	1202
	851	725	1576

Average household size	Chamars	4.46
" " "	Balars	4.43
" " "	All others	8.35

1901 Imperial Gazetteer of India to the large proportion of labourers in the population of Saharanpur district. There is, however, little information on the subject.) Importantly, also, the majority of landholdings are medium-sized. There are thus few landholdings larger than 8 or 10 acres.

The household sizes shown in Table 6.3 are of importance. Average household size among the Chamars and Balars, it will be noticed, is considerably smaller than it is among all other castes. This is due partly to the fact that there are more joint families among the better off households and partly because the number of children per couple (especially among Muslim castes) is high. The significance of this is that households with medium-sized landholdings have a considerable supply of family labour. Their need for extra (hired) labour is thereby reduced or even eliminated.

The traditional occupation - according to caste principles - of Chamars is leatherworking. This particular group, however, has not done any such work for a considerable period and regards itself as superior to other groups that do. Until the 1920s the principal occupations of the Chamars were agriculture and agricultural labour. From then onwards they began regularly to supplement their incomes by making rope. There is evidence to show that over the years landholdings became smaller and were finally lost - through uneconomic size, indebtedness or other factors. Thus individual households tended more and more towards landlessness, increasingly deriving their incomes through paid work and rope-making.

The situation among the Chamars today reflects this trend. There are a handful of households which live off their land alone, additionally making some rope when time permits; others which till their own land but also work for wages and make rope; and the majority, which lives entirely on rope-making and wage employment. The histories of many families, as well as the mere existence of the intermediate category, point to an ongoing process of change culminating in landlessness and in an expanding labour force.

Until about six years ago most families lived on what they earned through rope-making and wage labour in Mulkipur. At that point a combination of three factors led to their beginning temporary migration to other regions for work: inflation, which drastically reduced the buying power of their almost static incomes from the above two sources; decreasing demand for agricultural labour in Mulkipur; and increased demand for external labour in parts of Haryana and Punjab.

Inflation in India has been severe in recent years and the Chamars were badly affected. The real value of income from rope-making declined as the various middlemen involved succeeded in maintaining the absolute value of their cut, thus leaving the Chamars - who do the actual work - to face a rising price level without increased incomes. And agricultural wages in Mulkipur rose negligibly - their value fell considerably if seen in relation to prices.

Among households owning land in Mulkipur there was a steady decrease in per capita landholding; or, to put this in a manner relevant to the present argument, an increase in family labour available for agricultural tasks. I am not trying to argue that all of a sudden there was a slump in the wage employment offered by such households. Such a process is naturally a gradual one. But while for a time the Chamars could balance their decreasing income from wages by making more rope, and thus earning more, they could no longer manage this in the face of severe inflation.

The two factors discussed above show how a stage was reached when the Chamars' earnings within Mulkipur became insufficient to meet their needs. What led them to begin undertaking temporary work in Haryana and Punjab was the increased demand for external labour in those regions - expressing itself in greater availability of work as well as higher wages.

As is well known, Punjab State has shown the greatest improvement in agricultural productivity through increased use of new technology. The 'Green Revolution' was most successful there, primarily in terms of wheat production but significantly (although less publicised, since wheat has always been north India's most critical crop) also in production of other crops such as groundnuts. The following brief account of the factors leading to increased demand for external labour is based on Ludhiana district but applies generally to Punjab with the exception of the western districts of the state.

Before the 'Green Revolution' - intensive irrigation, use of chemical fertilisers and high-yielding varieties of seed, and some degree of mechanisation - most agriculture in Punjab followed the single-cropping pattern (except where canal water was available in abundance). In any one season some land was fallow and there was plenty of time to plough and manure it in preparation for the next season's sowing.

Thus at any time there was only one season's crop to be attended to, and even the busy seasons were not excessively so. The 'Green Revolution', bringing in its wake double - even treble - cropping, changed all this. Immediately a crop is harvested the land has to be prepared for the next sowing. The longer maturing periods of high-yielding varieties accentuates this problem. In sum, at least twice every year a great many tasks have to be crammed into a short period - harvesting (including threshing, sorting, storing, marketing, etc.), ploughing, manuring/fertilising, sowing, initial irrigation, and weeding. The care of a productive crop takes a good deal of work throughout the year but exceedingly intense labour in such peak periods.

In Punjab considerable development of industry and expansion of urban areas have also taken place. In addition to heavy industry the middle and small industrial sectors have grown rapidly since the state first started prospering. In consequence employment opportunities have increased substantially and, as is usually the case in such situations, a good deal of the agrarian labour force has been absorbed into the growing urban-industrial sector. Further, prosperity has led to a need for artisans in construction work, and mechanisation to a need for repair and maintenance facilities. Most families of landless labour in Punjab now have one or more members working outside the agricultural sector. The number of labourers available for agricultural work has therefore fallen significantly. In many villages it is not sufficient even to deal with regular slack-season activities. In all cases it is far short of peak-season demand. Thus two factors - increased work and intensity of work occasioned by the 'Green Revolution', and draining away of labour into urban-industrial employment - have combined to generate a great demand for external labour in Punjab in peak seasons.

A further factor is the prevalence of fertility control in Punjab. This leads to a reduction in family labour available to landowners, and also to a slower rate of growth of landless labourers' families.

The situation in Haryana is somewhat different. Demand for labour is restricted to paddy transplanting. In the areas to which the Mulkipur Chamars went it seems that a combination of mechanisation and relatively abundant local labour cause this. Wages here are lower than they are in Punjab.

Having discussed briefly the reasons for this high demand for external labour in Punjab and - less so - Haryana, we may look at some aspects of the migration proper.

One of the most important factors involved in migration is awareness of the availability of work and of workers on the part of labour and employers, respectively - in practical terms, the contact between employers and labour. In the case of the Chamars of Mulkipur, this is done by one or other of the following means: the employer or his representative comes either to Mulkipur or to the nearest town; the employer informs labour by post of the date the work is to begin, its duration, the number of people needed and the wages to be paid; a visiting labour party agrees to return on a roughly specified date to do the next job of work; a party of labour goes to Punjab or Haryana knowing only that work will be available somewhere in a certain cluster of villages.

The first and last of these methods are by far the most frequently seen. In the first case the employer usually gives a cash advance to cover travelling and other expenses, which also serves - importantly - to ensure that those who accept it will keep their word. The other method is adopted mainly by the younger people (for whom the work includes a component of adventure, and who do not feel as compelled as the older people to be absolutely certain in advance)but is frequently combined with the third-mentioned means, prior arrangement.

Minimal housing and sleeping facilities are provided by employers. In some cases one-way fare is also paid. In general, employers, while naturally striving to extract as much work as possible at the lowest expense, try to be pleasant, at least at the level of formality. When his own work is done an employer will find work elsewhere (nearby) for the visiting party, but, in view of the intense seasonal demand for labour, this is a favour to the next employer (usually a relative or friend) and not to the labourers.

Work is undertaken either on a daily wage basis or on piece rate terms (a certain area of land to be harvested, weeded, etc.). Labourers tend to prefer the latter system as this allows them to work the hours they like without constant goading from their employer. In general they earn more money in fewer days by putting in more hours of work per day. Employers also prefer it for this reason, and ensure that the work done is up to their standards by visiting the fields from time to time. Seen in terms of wages per hour worked the two systems are almost identical; the time factor is what decisions are based on.

Table 6.4 gives a breakdown of the migrant population by sex and age. Men of Mulkipur go to work in Punjab throughout the year. The only time that the village women also go is in the paddy transplanting season. There are two reasons for this. First, paddy transplanting is the only work in which female labour is specifically required. Second, since this is the only time that schoolgoing children can be taken along, it is effectively the only season when women can leave Mulkipur. Thus we find that the Chamar women of Mulkipur work only in Haryana while men work in Punjab as well. In Punjab food is provided by the employer; it is generally better and more substantial than that eaten in Mulkipur and therefore forms an important consideration for the labourers. In Haryana labourers are responsible for their own diet. The women take most of what they need - cooking utensils, spices and salt - along. Grain, vegetables, etc., are purchased at the place of work, often from the employer at prevailing market prices.

The importance of seasonal work outside Mulkipur can be seen from the figures given in Table 6.5. No less than 47 of the 70 Chamar households have one or more members working outside seasonally. These include households with up to 20 bighas of land. For almost all, the reason for beginning (and for continuing) to go to Punjab for work was debt. Without this supplementary income existence in Mulkipur had become impossible.

This particular form of migration has been in existence in the region for about six years. All the villages in the north of Saharanpur district send out such migrants seasonally; other villages, down to Muzaffarnagar and Meerut districts, also do so but to a lesser extent. The factors that have led to the need

TABLE 6.4

Subdivision of migrant population by sex and age*

Age group	Males	Females	Total	Percentage of age-group total
10-14	1	0	1	3.45
15-19	8	2	10	47.61
20-24	7	0	7	28.00
25-29	11	7	18	62.06
30-34	8	4	12	48.00
35-39	6	4	10	55.55
40-44	2	3	5	31.25
45-49	3	7	10	50.00
50-54	11	2	13	72.22
55-59	6	0	6	66.66
60-64	2	1	3	33.33
65+	1	0	1	6.66
Totals	66	30	96	41.02

* These figures refer only to working migrants. Children who are taken along but are too young to work are not represented.

TABLE 6.5

Chamar households subdivided by sex of migrating member(s)

	Number	Percentage
Households in which nobody migrates	23	32.8
Households in which only males migrate	20	28.6
Households in which both sexes migrate	27	38.6
	70	100.00

among labourers to supplement their incomes by working outside their own region have not altered. There is thus every reason to believe that such seasonal migration will continue to increase so long as there is a demand for labour in not-too-distant places.

CHAPTER 7

UNDERDEVELOPMENT AND DECLINING FERTILITY IN A KANDYAN VILLAGE

Demographic theory has generally associated declining rates of fertility with the processes unleashed by economic development, i.e. a shift of a substantial proportion of the labour force from agriculture to industry, a rise in the real income of the people, urbanisation, the spreading of education and health facilities, disintegration of traditional family organisation and the increasing participation of women in industrial and service sectors. Historically, the gradual decline of fertility in Western Europe and North America and the sharp decline in Japan resulted precisely due to these processes. More recently, the islands of Taiwan, Singapore and Hong Kong have also been added to this group of societies, which experienced a decline in fertility due to economic development.

During the past one-and-a-half decades, Sri Lanka has also experienced a substantial decline in fertility. The crude birth rate, which was 37.0 in 1959, came down to 29.4 in 1970, and the downward trend seems to be continuing. The purpose of this essay is to argue that the decline in Sri Lanka is not related to economic development, but on the contrary, to a process that runs in the opposite direction, namely the perpetuation of underdevelopment.[1] The hypotheses advanced can be summarised in three points.

Firstly, the underdeveloped economy of Sri Lanka is incapable of creating sufficient employment opportunities for the young adults who are currently in the marriageable age groups. High rates of unemployment compel the young adults to depend on their

---

1. The word 'underdevelopment' is used here in the sense that it is employed in the works of Baran (1957), Frank (1969) *et al.* Underdevelopment is not a condition that existed in the 'Third World' countries prior to colonial domination. It is a condition created and perpetuated by the colonial powers on the basis of the transfer of resources to the metropolitan centres. Underdevelopment is mainly a process of uneven development, accumulation in the metropolis and stagnation in the hinterlands. In order to facilitate the resource transfer to the metropolitan centres, the service sector consisting of transport, communication, etc., has expanded to a certain degree in the hinterlands, which must not be taken as economic development. On the contrary, the societies subjected to resource transfer are not developing countries but underdeveloping countries. This uneven development is further documented in Chapter 8.

parents, which gives rise to a high dependency ratio. This raises the age at marriage and effectively reduces the most fertile period of a woman's child-bearing age, thus contributing to a general fertility decline.

Secondly, the general decline in marital fertility that pertains to all social classes is caused, in the final analysis, by the incapacity of the economy to absorb a growing number of labour units.

Finally, the differential decline of marital fertility, which indicates a lesser rate of decline among the poor, is related on the whole to the condition of underdevelopment.

I will attempt to substantiate these hypotheses primarily in relation to data obtained from the village of Delumgoda, which is located in the Udunwara Revenue Officers division, Kandy District, and is about 11 miles away from Kandy, the district capital. Whenever necessary, supplementary nation-wide data will be presented.

The social history of villages such as Delumgoda is invariably linked with the structural changes occurring in the country as a whole. The introduction of the plantations, the resultant expansion of the roads to serve them and the accompanying growth of towns as commercial centres exercised a dominative influence over the Kandyan villages from the mid-19th century. The forces unleashed by these structural changes were manifold, and reacted on the structure and further reinforced the changes that were taking place. For example, part of the land was claimed by the colonial state and was sold to the British companies to be turned into large scale plantations. The ancestral lands held by the peasant families were converted into commodities sold in the market, thus always tending to alienate the poorest groups of peasants from the land that ancestrally belonged to them. In agriculture, the surplus product became a commodity that could be sold in the market. This led to the increasing commercialisation of agriculture and the worsening of the condition of the rural poor, who could not rely on the village grain surplus any more.

As a result of the expansion of commodity production, the exchange relations became mainly monetised. Whenever money penetrates a traditional economy, where barter used to be the predominant traditional form, it has a tendency to reify the exchange relations and set them against those social relations on which the traditional social order was based. Commodity production and the monetisation of exchange logically implies that the village economy gets increasingly absorbed into the national structure, and through it inevitably into the world economy. In consumption, as well as in production inputs, the village becomes an organic but dependent part of the national and the global economy. Working for a wage, where the actual producer is alienated from the means of production, emerges in the countryside as an important production relation. This new form of employment - as against the old forms, such as labour rent *(Rajakariya)*, exchange labour *(attam)* and share-cropping *(ande)* - reduces the content of the social relationship between the employer and the employee into a mere cash nexus and disrupts the traditional social fabric.

All these processes, with their attendant disruption of the traditional social relations, can be seen at work in Delumgoda, where 90 acres of land bordering the adjoining village of Hiddaula was claimed by the colonial state and converted into a tea plantation in the late 19th century. This reduced the potential land area in which the village could have expanded, although it also provided employment for some of the village poor. Buying and selling of land started in the mid-19th century, alienating the poor from the land and tending to further concentrate the land in the hands of the affluent. The land records are full of instances of mortgage, lease and outright sale. For example, a single non-resident family group owns 19 acres of paddy land and over 50 acres of highland. 55.7% of the heads of households in the village do not own any paddy land. Nearly half of them, however, possess cultivation rights since they work as share-croppers for various landlords. 69% of the households do not own any highland (defined as non-irrigated land excluding house and garden). The ownership of houses is more widespread, with only 19% of the heads of households having no legal title to their houses.

Agriculture, especially in the past decade, has become definitely market-oriented. The old division between commercial crops and subsistence crops no longer holds. Rice, the subsistence staple par excellence, has also become a major commercial crop. Even the poorest share-croppers, who do not produce enough rice for their own subsistence, sell their grain in the market. The bulk of the produce going to the market, however, comes from the affluent landlords.

In exchange relations, with the exception of that between the share-cropper and the landlord, money dominates. The villagers have become consumers inextricably linked with the national market. Barter has disappeared, except in those cases where it represents a monetary relation in content. In production as well as consumption, Delumgoda has become integrated into the global economy. All the cultivators in Delumgoda use modern high-yielding varieties of paddy, which require expensive inputs such as fertiliser and insecticide. The extent of mechanisation is very limited. In spite of this, paddy agriculture has become increasingly dependent on the inputs coming from outside. In consumption too, the villagers are heavily dependent on the commodities coming from outside - rice, flour, oil, sugar, clothes, manufactured products, etc.

The employment structure also indicates the increasing integration with the national economy. 21% of the heads of households (consisting of school teachers, supervisors and urban workers) are employed on a regular basis in the modern sector and earn monthly salaries.

TABLE 7.1

Population growth and paddy cultivated area in Delumgoda

	1881	1891	1901	1911	1921	1931	1946	1953	1963	1974
Population	228	186	223	255	254	335	370	417	513	683
Paddy land in acres	37.5	38.5	-	-	-	-	-	-	43	43
Paddy Land per capita	.16	.20	-	-	-	-	-	-	.08	.06

Sources: Census Reports, unpublished records of the Department of Census and Statistics and Lawrie (1896:358).

In the period 1901-1974, the population of Delumgoda increased threefold. In the inter-census period 1946-1953, the rate of increase was 12.7%; the growth rate for the decade 1953-1963 was 22.4%; and the highest growth rate was for the 11-year period 1963-1974, which was 33.0%. The very high growth rate for the 1963-1974 period is not entirely due to the maintenance of high fertility rates, but primarily to migration into the village. A number of landless families from the adjoining village of Rabbegamuwa moved into the village and occupied some land owned by the government in the relevant period. The declining fertility trend emerges, however, from the age pyramid (Chart 7.1). The age cohort 10-14 is the largest with 87 persons, followed by the age cohort 5-9 consisting of 81 persons. The drop is sharp in the 0-4 age cohort, which includes only 64 individuals.

The paddy cultivated area has remained nearly static since 1891. It is possible that the slight increase indicated in Table 7.1 is due to better recording methods, rather than to any actual increase in the paddy acreage. The shift from single cropping to double cropping, which occurred nearly 20 years ago and the application of labour-intensive methods, such as transplanting, adopted more recently, would have definitely made the village economy capable of absorbing more labour units than it did earlier. But the labour absorption capacity of agriculture, in paddy cultivation or in the cultivation of other crops, is necessarily limited. Delumgoda would have passed the capacity for providing employment for all members of the village labour force, in agriculture and related occupations, at least two decades ago.

The primarily agrarian economy of Delumgoda becomes incapable of supporting the growing population, which is a result of the historically-maintained high fertility rates supplemented

CHART 7.1

Delumgoda 1974: age/sex pyramid

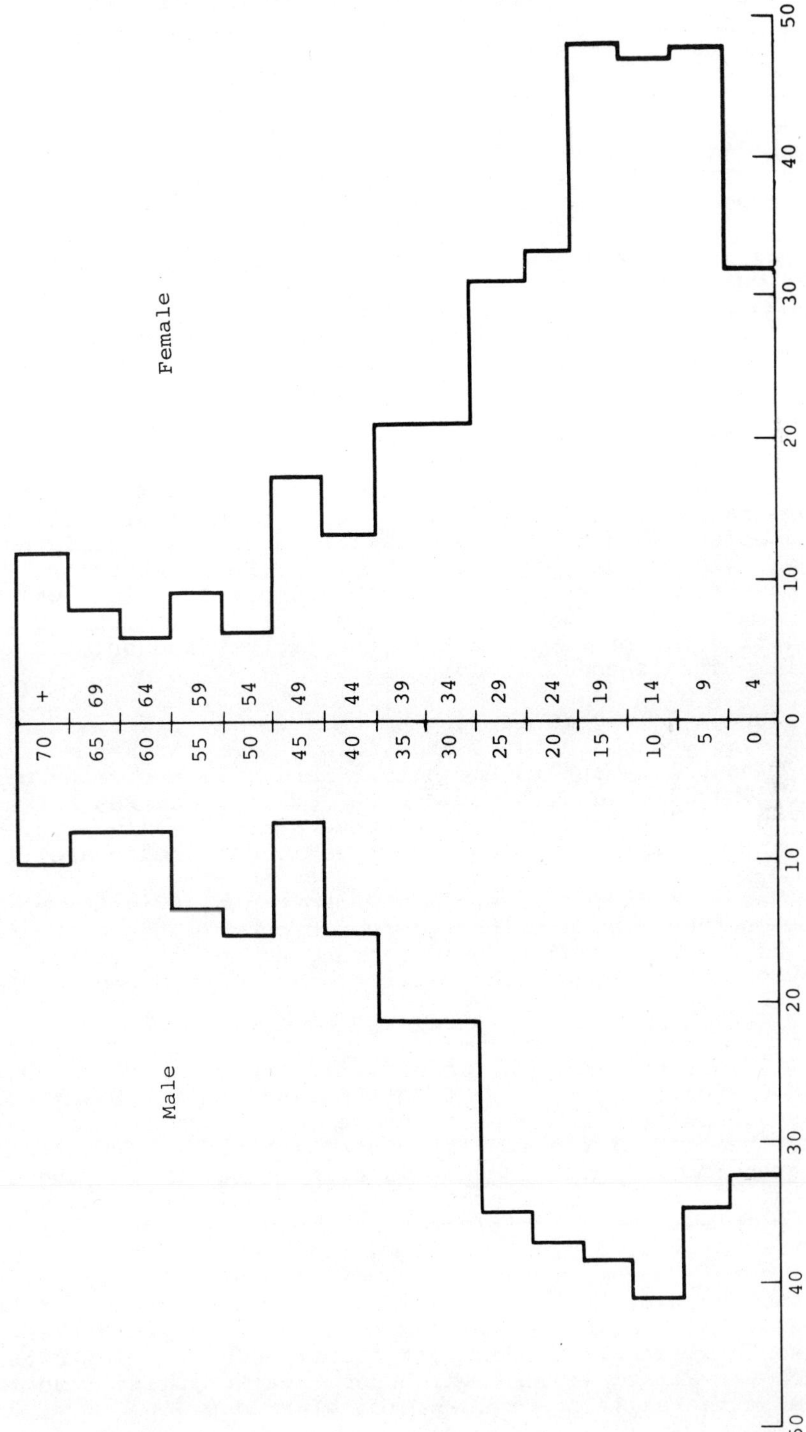

by the declining mortality rates. If the members of the labour force are to be employed, it becomes imperative to create employment opportunities in the non-agrarian sector, either within or outside the village. Such a programme would require a high degree of capital accumulation, which in the last analysis rests on the amount of the surplus extracted and the ways in which it is disposed of. Baran (1957) has demonstrated the availability of two varieties of surplus in underdeveloped countries: the actual surplus and the potential surplus.

Part of the actual surplus is directly exported to the international metropolitan centres and the rest is conspicuously consumed by the upper classes. The potential surplus, however, is never realised due to the irrational nature of the social organisation of production.[2] The perpetuation of underdevelopment thus makes it impossible for a country to create sufficient employment for its labour force, which could only be created in the non-agrarian sector.

A step in the right direction, however, was made when a powerloom factory, administered by the Department of Small Industries, was established in Delumgoda. The factory primarily depends on female labour and employs 120 women. But the factory recruits labour from the entire Udunuwara Revenue Division, which had a population of 66,368 in 1971. As a result, there was great competition to get employment in the factory and only 12 women from Delumgoda succeeded in doing so.

Though Delumgoda is located only 11 miles from Kandy, the unemployed young adults of the village find it extremely difficult to find employment in the city. Kandy, like so many cities in the 'Third World', is not a manufacturing centre, but a centre of circulation. As an administrative and commercial nucleus, the amount of employment opportunities it can create are limited.

The insufficient employment opportunities in the non-agrarian sector thus emerge as the basic factor related to the prevalance of high rates of unemployment among the young adults. The gravity of the problem is heaviest among the educated youth (defined

---

2. A share-cropper who obtains his inputs (seed paddy, insecticides, fertiliser, etc.) from the landlord can be cited as a case in point. Since he is compelled to pay 50% of the produce and the cost of the inputs to the landlord after harvest, the share-cropper does not show much interest in applying all the inputs. It may be more profitable, from his point of view, to sell them to some other cultivator on the black market. I have come across several disputes between landlords and share-croppers which resulted from such sales of inputs. If every cultivator owned the plot that he cultivated and was not obliged to pay rents, this would be unlikely to occur, and the harvest would also be greater. The concept of potential surplus refers to such unrealised wealth, which does not actualise itself precisely due to the existing organisation of production.

as those who have completed their GCE 'O' Level). This does not, however, imply that the less-educated youth have sufficient employment opportunities. Some of them in Delumgoda have become seasonally migrant agricultural workers, travelling 70 miles or more to the North Central Province where the wages are high during the peak periods of the agricultural cycle. In the village context they can only hope for casual employment, which means being idle for 10 to 15 days per month. The young adult, especially in the rural lower middle classes, often continues to be dependent on his parents well into her/his late 20s. Among the mid-peasants, the young adult may help his parents in working the land, but if he is educated - which he often is - he would not take cultivation as a 'job'. Among the poor peasants and the rural workers the degree of dependence of young adults on the parents is lesser than in other classes, but it is by no means absent.

TABLE 7.2

Age-specific marital statistics in Delumgoda, 1974

	Total No.	Male No.	Female No.	Married*		Never married	
				Male %	Female %	Male %	Female %
15-19	86	38	48	0.0	2.0	100.0	98.0
20-24	70	37	33	5.4	18.1	94.6	81.9
25-29	65	34	31	39.4	58.0	60.6	42.0
30-34	42	21	21	47.6	71.4	52.4	28.6
35-39	42	21	21	71.4	90.4	28.6	9.6
40-44	28	15	13	86.6	92.3	13.4	7.7
45-49	25	7	18	85.7	100.0	14.3	0.0

* includes persons divorced and widowed.

Turning now to the possible causes of the general decline in marital fertility, it is evident from Tables 7.2 and 7.3 that 98.0% of the women in the age cohort 15-19 are unmarried. Even in the age group 20-24, the marital rate does not change significantly and about 82% of the women are unmarried. 42% of women continue to be unmarried in the age cohort 25-29 as well. Only in the age cohort 30-34 does the rate change significantly, with only 28.6% being unmarried.

TABLE 7.3

Proportions of women never married by age group for Sri Lanka, the relevant zone and Delumgoda

	Sri Lanka		Zone*		Delumgoda
	1963	1970	1963	1970	1974
15-19	85.0	91.3	85.1	92.8	98.0
20-24	41.3	56.1	36.3	58.3	81.9
25-29	17.1	22.9	12.8	19.2	42.0
30-34	8.3	9.0	5.8	5.3	28.6
35-39	4.8	5.0	3.4	3.0	9.6
40-44	4.3	2.8	3.2	2.2	7.7
45-49	3.9	2.3	2.6	2.1	0.0

* The relevant zone consists of Kandy, Matale, Nuwara Eliya, Badulla, Ratnapura, Kegalle and Kurunegala Districts

Source for statistics on Sri Lanka and the Zone: Fernando (1974).

The data that pertains to the island and the relevant zone indicates a number of important trends.

Firstly, the overwhelming majority of women in the age group 15-19 are unmarried; a substantial proportion of them get married in the age group 20-24, but still more than half of them continue to be unmarried. In the age group 25-29, nearly 80% of them are married and the proportion of unmarried women significantly declines thereafter.

Secondly, a comparison of figures for 1963 and 1970 indicates an increase in the proportion of unmarried women in all the three relevant age cohorts in between 15-29. In the relevant zone there had been a sharp increase in the age cohort 20-24. The proportion went up from 36.3% in 1963 to 58.3% in 1970.

The village data indicate more or less the same tendency, i.e. a very high proportion of unmarried women in the age group 15-29. They vary however from the national and zonal figures, as the tendency is particularly pronounced in Delumgoda. Further, a comparatively higher proportion of women seem to remain unmarried, even in the age cohort 40-44. It is likely that this is due to a number of factors. For instance, the figures that pertain to the Zone include the population living on the plantations. The socio-economic structure and the cultural values among the plantation workers are quite distinct from those of the Kandyan villagers. In general, the plantation workers tend to marry early and it is possible that the data pertaining to them has raised the general proportion of married women. Further, it is evident from the zonal figures that the rate of increase of the proportion of unmarried women in the age group 20-24 between 1963 and 1970 is 22%. If one assumes a linear trend, by 1974 the proportion would have increased to 70.9%, which is closer to the proportion of women unmarried in Delumgoda. Finally, the Kandyan areas are hinterland communities, in relation to the coastal areas in the Western Province. The process of underdevelopment is most pronounced here. Since employment opportunities in the non-agrarian sector are least available in the Kandyan villages, the proportions of women unmarried also may be high.

The nation-wide increase in the proportion of women unmarried has also been explained in relation to purely demographic factors. Fernando (1975), for instance, has attributed it to an imbalance in the sex ratio of the corresponding age cohorts. Thus in 1971, there were only 81.1 males per 100 females (relevant age cohorts being 15-29 for females and 20-34 for males). The figures for Delumgoda are comparable; for 100 females in the age cohort 15-29, there are 82.1 males in the 20-34 age cohort. No doubt this imbalance has contributed to the problem, but nevertheless it does not causally explain its existence. If the problem is entirely due to the imbalance, one would expect a higher proportion of males in the relevant age cohort to be married. In Delumgoda, in the age cohort 20-34, 23.9% of men are married; by comparison, in the age cohort 19-29, 22.3% of women are married. The difference is too marginal to warrant an explanation based on an imbalance of the sex ratio.

TABLE 7.4

Average number of children ever born per currently married women by age group and social class in Delumgoda, 1974

	15-24	25-34	35-44	45-54
Class I	0	1.6	5.0	6.0
Class II	0	2.2	4.0	6.2
Class III	1.0	3.6	7.2	8.1
Class IV	0	1.3	5.5	7.0
Class V	1.0	3.9	5.7	10.0

If a purely demographic analysis does not yield an adequate explanation for the observed general decline in marital fertility, it becomes necessary to consider other possible reasons. At the same time it will be seen that there is a differential decline according to social class. Data from Table 7.4 will be used to illustrate these points, with the aid of representative case studies drawn from each social class.

Class I consists of teachers, supervisory workers and other salaried white collar employees who are often land owners. In this class, the age at marriage is high. The young women, whose parents hold the above positions, are forced by social values to get married to males with regular employment and a monthly salary. The bridegrooms of this stratum expect a dowry, especially if the woman is unemployed. This creates problems, particularly in those families with a number of daughters. The marital fertility rate in this stratum is also comparatively low. The parents expect their children to complete at least their secondary education. They also tend to attend the better schools located outside the village, which implies daily commuting by bus. Moreover, the children of this stratum do no agricultural work. They start earning only in the mid 20s. The benefits coming from the state welfare system are more than off-set by the heavy expenditure involved. The members of this class are strongly motivated by an ideology of social mobility. Seen in terms of this ideology, a large family, even where parents are capable of maintaining one, does not make much sense.

Case A. MGJ, a school teacher, is 35 years of age. He was born to a family of land-holding cultivators and attended a government school six miles away from the village. He joined the Education Department as a teacher, after completing his secondary education, and entered a teachers' training college later. He married MA, also a school-teacher, whom he met at the teachers' training college. It is a cross-caste union. Their joint income in the form of salaries received, is in excess of Rs. 750.00 per month. MGJ has not yet inherited the land due to him from his father, as the latter is still alive. Last year he purchased half an acre of paddy land, which is given out for share-cropping. He obtains around 40 bushels of paddy per annum as his share.

MGJ married five years ago, when he was 30 years of age; his wife was then 27 years old. They have two children, a boy aged four and a girl aged two. He would like to have another child, but not as yet. He is also thinking of moving closer to Kandy when his children grow up. MGJ is aware of family planning techniques, but has relied mainly on natural methods. No child of this family has died in infancy.

Class II consists of owner-cultivators who are not compelled to sell their labour. They own plots of paddy land and highland which provide them with a sufficient income to maintain their way of life. In this social class, too, the age at marriage is comparatively high. The younger members of this class are also education-oriented, but their chances of getting employment are not as high as those of the former class. Their parents do not possess the same influence as those of Class I in rural society, to find them employment.[3] When they become employed in the modern sector they tend to get less prestigious jobs in spite of their educational accomplishments. In seeking partners, the young women of this class are not entirely motivated to find one with regular employment and a monthly salary. But they are unlikely to marry a rural worker with no land. The marital fertility in this class is *lower* than that of Class I, but is *higher* than the rate that pertains to the poor peasants and the rural workers. The children of this class are not as alienated from agriculture as those of the former class; they help their parents. But the economic benefit gained from this loses its significance due to the money that has to be spent on their education.

Case B. DMD (aged 40) is an owner-cultivator, who owns a home garden one acre in extent, an acre of paddy land and two acres of highland. In addition, he has leased on a money rent basis half an acre of paddy land. He also owns a small building where a shop used to be located, but now he derives no income from this, as there is no tenant. His monthly income from land exceeds Rs. 400.00 per month.

He was 27 years old when he married DMS, who was then 23 years old. They have five children, two boys and three girls. Their age distribution is as follows; 12, 10, 8, 4 and 8 months. The three elder children attend the school located in the village. The spacing of children, especially in the case of the younger three, indicates that DMD is conscious of the problem of having too many children.

DMD thinks that it is better to have sons than daughters. In fact, he had been expecting a son this time, when the baby girl was born. Though he is aware of family planning methods, he believes that the force of *Karma*[4] operates in deciding the number and the sex of children. The two boys aged 12 and 10 help their

---

3. The state is the major employer in Sri Lanka's modern sector. Recruitment into these much-sought-after positions in the state and the semi-state sector, *de jure* occurs on the basis of merit. However, in the *de facto* recruitment procedure, political influence plays a highly important role. A recommendation from the local representative to the State Assembly is thought to be necessary to obtain many jobs in the state sector. Only the people with sufficient influence in rural society are capable of getting these recommendations.

4. Buddhism teaches that every volitional action has its result which may come to one either in this life or in the later-lives. *Karma* is the force that is attributed to these actions, which one has committed in past births or in the past of the present birth. Good volitional actions are capable of giving good results i.e. birth in an exalted position and well being, while bad actions cause birth in an inferior position and much suffering. Thus both fortune and misfortune can be explained in terms of the *Karma* theory.

father in agriculture, performing less demanding tasks. But DMD would prefer them to have jobs in the modern sector when they grow up. DMS has obtained family planning advice from the midwife. No child in this family has died in infancy.

Class III consists of poor peasants, defined as those who either own small plots of land or who are share-croppers. All the poor peasants obtain an income from land, but they are compelled to sell their labour to supplement it. The age at marriage is slightly lower than in the case of the former two classes. The young members of this class are not as education-oriented as those in I and II. They attend the village schools but often drop out before completing their secondary education. When someone from this stratum completes his secondary education, he is less likely to find a job in the modern sector. Thus the possibility of marrying early among the young, who primarily consist of secondary school drop-outs, depends on the labour requirements that the agrarian sector can generate. The sons of this stratum are unlikely to inherit sufficient land from their parents to depend on owner-cultivation. The double process of fragmentation of land and population growth drives the young members of this class towards unskilled irregular employment. The marital fertility rate is comparatively high, since the investment the children require is less. In this stratum the children also help their parents in cultivation. They would have earned money if the demand for unskilled labour had been high. But Delumgoda does not provide enough opportunities in that direction.

The state social welfare system also emerges as an important variable influencing the fertility patterns of this class. The welfare system could be manipulated to suit the necessities of a family living at the bare subsistence level. In Sri Lanka, everyone who does not pay income tax (children as well as adults) receives 1lb of rice per week free of charge, and another two pounds at a special subsidised price. The ration card also entitles these people to various other commodities, such as dried fish, sugar, clothes etc. At the poorest level, the food habits of the villagers change and rice becomes a luxury. Some of the free rice obtained from the co-operative store is sold and the money is used to buy bread and yam. The ration card entitles everyone to ¾lb sugar per month. The price of sugar in the black market varies between Rs. 8.00 and Rs. 10.00. It is possible to sell a pound of sugar for Rs. 7.00 to a pedlar and one spends only 72 cents in buying it. If one had seven childrent, one would have nine ration cards and by selling sugar alone one would earn Rs. 54.00, which is more than the wages of the head of the household for 10 days.

But even in this class marital fertility is slowly declining, which must be related to the general lack of employment opportunities. The rate of infant mortality is high in this class and life expectancy is comparatively low.

Case C. HGS (aged 45) is a share-cropper who cultivates a plot of paddy land half an acre in extent. In addition, he also cultivates a half-acre plot owned by the temple of Lankatilaka and pays labour rent in the form of carrying the insignia of the deity in the annual temple procession. The landlord charges the cost of the inputs which he advances, plus 50% of the produce. From paddy cultivation and wage labour, HGS earns around Rs. 200.00 a month. His eldest son contributes another Rs. 60.00 to Rs. 80.00 to the family coffers.

HGS married VGHM (now aged 40), in 1952. It is a *Binna*(uxorilocal) union and the woman is his cross-cousin. VGHM gave birth to eight children but one of them died in infancy. The age distribution of the surviving children is as follows; 21, 19, 17, 15, 13, 10 and 6. None of the children are married. The three elder children are secondary school drop-outs. The younger children, except the one aged 6 are currently attending the village school. The elder children help the parents in agricultural activities.

HGS has not invested very much in his children. In fact, they have become economic assets to a certain degree, as they help him in agriculture, earn some money and also become valuable aids to manipulating the state social welfare system. But the children would have been of greater benefit if HGS held more land, and/or if employment opportunities in the agrarian sector were readily available. Since this is not the case even in the poor peasant stratum, the rationality that was once attached to having a large family is gradually being eroded.

Class IV consists of urban workers who are resident in the village. They generally come from the owner-cultivator families and are employed in the urban areas as watchers, peons, drivers etc. The majority of the urban workers own land in the village, which accounts for their continued residence there. Generally, they enjoy living standards superior to the poor peasants and the agrarian workers.

As far as value orientations are concerned, they are closer to Class I than to any other agrarian stratum. An ideology of social mobility pervades this stratum; those who are blue-collar workers are interested in pushing their children in to the white-collar stratum. Hence, education becomes an important field of investment. The majority of them, however, cannot afford to send their children to the prestigious urban schools. The children of this class attend either the village schools or the government secondary schools located near to the village.

The girls of this class are interested in getting married to a man with a monthly salary and regular employment, even if he is a blue-collar worker. This raises the age at marriage and the proportion of young women unmarried in this category is high. Marital fertility in this class is closer to that of Class I. Since the urban workers are less agriculture-oriented than workers in the other agrarian strata, children are not so important to them as labour units in agriculture.

Case D. DGW (aged 38) is a Police-constable, attached to the Kandy Police Station. He commutes for work daily. He owns half an acre of paddy land, a house and a garden. The paddy plot is cultivated by means of wage labour and he obtains approximately 50 bushels of paddy per annum. His salary is Rs. 400.00.

He married LGB (now aged 36) from Kandy, seven years ago. They have three children, two boys and a girl, respectively aged 6, 4 and 1. None of the children are yet old enough to attend school. PGW is conscious of the burden of having a large family. When his children grow up he will have to invest in their education. Moreover, since the land owned is cultivated by wage labour, the children are not important as labour units.

DGW is practising modern family planning methods; he obtained advice from a doctor attached to a rural maternity hospital six miles away. No child in this family has died in infancy.

Class V consists of rural labourers who possess no rights over productive land and who depend entirely on income from wages for their sustenance. This excludes the share-croppers and temple tenants who possess some form of right over land. The members of this class are rural labourers, who work in the paddy fields and the high land. They are also engaged in various unskilled tasks such as carrying weights and assisting skilled workers of certain categories. Their employment is of an irregular nature and they are fully employed only at the peaks of the agricultural cycle. The paucity of demand for their labour in the village has driven them to become migrant workers and some of them travel to the North Central Province in the planting and harvesting seasons.

In their value orientation they are not very different from the poor peasants. Their children attend only the primary school and many of them drop out. Though the Government schools do not charge fees, the cost involved in buying books and dressing the children properly is exorbitant in comparison to their income. The investment in children is low. On the contrary, just as in the case of the poor peasantry, in manipulating the social welfare system the children become valuable assets. Hence, the marital fertility rate is high.

The age at marriage is comparatively low in this class. A girl cannot expect to marry a man with regular employment or a land-owning cultivator. Dowries are neither expected nor given. As soon as a young man is capable of getting regular employment, if he has no major obligations to his parents and siblings, he is in a position to get married and generally does so.

Case E. KMA (aged 41) is a rural labourer. He owns no land; the hut which he occupies stands on a plot of land owned by an aristocratic land-owning family. He does not pay a monetary rent, but he is expected to work on his landlord's fields in the peak seasons without payment. He undertakes any irregular employment that comes his way, both agricultural as well as non-agricultural. When he works on the paddy fields, he receives

Rs. 5.00 per day plus tea and snacks. He is not given food when he works on the high land or when he is engaged in non-agricultural unskilled work. Mostly piece rates prevail and the wage is negotiated. His wife, TGB (aged 38), also works for wages when she can find work, which generally happens in the peak periods of the paddy cultivation cycle. She earns Rs. 3.00 to Rs. 4.00 per day.

KMA married TGB in 1955 when they were respectively aged 22 and 19. She came from Delumgoda itself and is a classificatory cross-cousin of KMA. TGB gave birth to nine children but one died in infancy. The age distribution of the remaining eight children is as follows: 18, 12, 10, 8, 6, 5, 4 and 1. The two elder daughters did not attend school. The son aged 10 attended primary school but dropped out after completing only Grade II.

The grown-up girl does not earn any money, but spends her time looking after her younger siblings. KMA thinks that the number and the sex of the children is decided by *Karma*. But he is more concerned with the sex of the children than with their number. If his first-born had been a son, now he would be in a position to lessen his father's burden. His second-born was a son, but he died due to KMA's *Karma*. KMA is aware of family planning methods, but is not convinced of the benefits that these methods could bring him.

Conclusion

The decline of fertility in Sri Lanka is directly associated with two factors: very high proportions of unmarried women in the 15-29 age group, and a general decline in the marital fertility rate. In a social system where pre-marital sex is highly disapproved of, the fertility of these unmarried women is near to zero, which contributes to the fertility decline of the general population in a most significant way. I demonstrated the causal relationship between the high proportions of unmarried women and the underdeveloped economy, which is incapable of generating sufficient employment opportunities. The decline in the marital fertility trend has two observable features. Firstly, the rate has declined in relation to all classes, which partly results from the declining rates of infantile mortality, and partly from the low capacity of the economy to absorb labour, which reduces the importance of the children as labour units. Secondly, the differential rate of decline in relation to various classes results from the operation of secondary variables, such as the high investment in children which the affluent engage in and the manipulation of the welfare system on which the poor rely.

The declining rate of fertility in Sri Lanka cannot be explained in terms of the standard demographic transition theory, which assumes sustained economic development as its base. The service sector in Sri Lanka, the transport system, the communication network, the education and health services have definitely made some advances. But this expansion is heavily service-oriented, which implies that the bulk of the population are still engaged in the agrarian sector and their real income has remained static or is even decreasing. The expansion of the service sector is not a sign of economic development but a structural incongruity of the economy which in itself is a facet of underdevelopment. Sri Lanka demonstrates that even the perpetuation of underdevelopment, given a certain degree of expansion of the service sector, can generate the necessary conditions for a decline in fertility.

CHAPTER 8

A SRI LANKAN VILLAGE ON THE VERGE OF A DEMOGRAPHIC TRANSITION

INTRODUCTION

As mentioned in the previous chapter, Sri Lanka has been experiencing a declining birth rate along with a rapid fall in mortality rates. For example the crude birth rate has changed from 35.7 per 1,000 in 1940, to 39.7 in 1950 and 29.4 in 1970. Similarly, the crude death rate declined from 22.0 per 1,000 in 1954, to 12.6 in 1950 and to 8.6 in 1960.

Even though similar data on the historical demographic pattern for Aluthgama-Bogamuwa[1] is not available, the age-sex distribution of the population - i.e. a low proportion of lower age groups 0-4, 5-9, clearly indicates a falling birth rate and changing fertility patterns over the past 15 years. The crude birth rate for the village in 1974 was 22.9 per 1,000, which is substantially lower than the equivalent national figure of 29.4 for 1971.

Here I try to examine not only the recent changes in the village's demographic trends, but also their reasons. I suggest that the decline in the birth rate is the result of a rising age at marriage and a reduction in marital fertility which in turn reflects the changes in the socio-economic structure and the introduction of welfare facilities (see p151). Estimated fertility for the total village population (see Table 8.1) and the age specific fertility rates indicate that it is a comparatively low fertility area. The village figures are much lower than the national estimates of age specific fertility

Life expectancy at birth for the village is comparatively high and similar to the national figures. Expected life at birth for the village population is between 66-68, which resembles the national figures given in Table 8.2

In Sri Lanka, the expectation of life at birth has improved rapidly since World War II as a result of better health facilities and slightly improved living standards, which were accompanied by a sharp decline in the rate of mortality among infants and child-bearing mothers. Infant mortality was reduced from 141 in 1946 to about 50 in 1968.

---

1. This is the Sri Lankan village which the author studied, and which provides the base data for the analysis presented in this chapter.

TABLE 8.1

Fertility data in Aluthgama-Bogamuwa

Age Group	No. of women enumerated	No. of mothers	Total live births	Mean parity	Total No. of births in previous year	Total No. of children dead	ASFR	d	Multiplying factors	ASFR for 1969 in Sri Lanka	q	t	l	Matching level	ASFR x 5 f	F	Central Age	ASFR x Cent.age	Multiplying factors	m. factors x f	F + kf A	B	B/A
15–19	100	2	3	0.03	2	0	0.020	0	1.129	.046	-	1	1		.100	-	17.5	.350	.268	.027	.027	.030	1.111
20–24	80	20	36	0.45	13	3	0.163	0.083	1.082	.212	.0898	2	.9102	70–75	.815	.100	22.5	3.668	.540	.440	.540	.450	.833
25–29	59	28	63	1.068	10	3	0.169	0.048	1.033	.250	.0496	3	.9504	85–90	.845	.915	27.5	4.648	.593	.501	1.416	1.068	.754
30–34	71	52	165	2.324	8	8	0.113	0.048	1.031	.191	.0495	5	.9505	90–95	.565	1.760	32.5	3.673	.624	.353	2.113	2.324	1.100
35–39	64	56	223	3.484	5	13	0.078	0.058	1.040	.138	.0603	10	.9397	90–95	.390	2.315	37.5	2.925	.649	.253	2.578	3.484	1.351
40–44	38	35	150	3.947	1	10	0.026	0.067	1.021	.040	.0684	15	.9316	90–95	.013	2.715	42.5	1.105	.702	.009	2.724	3.947	1.449
45–49	43	37	142	3.302	-	8	-	0.056	1.021	.006	.0572	20	.9428	95–100									
50–54	21	14	63	3.0	-	5	-	0.079	1.036		.0818	25	.9182	90–95				16.369					
55-59	36	28	122	3.389	-	16	-	0.131	1.039														
60–64	20	18	79	3.95	-	8	-	0.4															
65	43	39	88	-	-	20	-	0.227															
						Total:	0.569																

$$m = \frac{16.369}{.569} = 28.768$$

1^{o}_{o} = 66–68 years

TFR

(1) $\frac{(P3)^2}{P2} = 2.535$

(2) (P45-49) + 10% = 3.632

(3) $\frac{(P40\text{-}44) + (P45\text{-}49)}{2} + 10\% = 3.98$

TABLE 8.2

Life expectancy in Sri Lanka

Year	Males	Females
1910 - 12	33.4	29.3
1920 - 22	32.7	30.7
1945 - 47	46.8	44.7
1952	57.6	55.5
1965	63.7	65.0
1967	64.8	66.9

TABLE 8.3

Distribution of highland ownership and employment

		Employed household heads	
	Nos.	Nos.	%
1. Landless*	59	32	54
2. Less than ½ acre	87	41	47
3. ½ - less than 1 acre	60	24	40
4. 1 - less than 2½ acres	70	25	36
5. 2½- less than 5 acres	23	9	39
6. 5 - less than 10 acres	10	6	60
7. 10 acres and over	5	0	0

* Landlessness does not necessarily denote the lowest economic stratum. There are a number of families in the village who have no land but derive a considerable income fron non-agricultural sources.

TABLE 8.4

Distribution of income (annual) in the village

Income group	A) Households		B) In Migrated Households	
	Nos.	%	Nos.	B/A as a %
Less than Rs. 3,000	102	32	22	21
Rs. 3,000-7,000	122	39	34	28
Rs. 7,000-10,000	34	11	7	21
Rs. 10,000 and above	56	18	24	43
TOTAL	314	100	87	28

TABLE 8.5

Total fertility rates according to income group

Income Group	$\frac{(P3)^2}{P2}$	(P40-49) + 10%	Child/Woman Ratio (per 1,000 women) Pop. 0-4/Women 15-44
Less than Rs. 3,000	5.15	3.57	288
Rs. 3,000 - 7,000	2.265	3.57	402
Rs. 7,000 - 10,000	0.928	3.71	263
Rs.10,000 and above	-	3.28	194

TABLE 8.6

Mean parity (age specific) according to income category

Age Group \ Income Group	Less than Rs. 3,000	Rs. 3,000 to Rs. 7,000	Rs. 7,000 to Rs. 10,000	Rs. 10,000 & above
15-19	0.033	0.069	-	-
20-24	0.583	0.594	0.333	-
25-29	1.733	1.16	0.556	0.429
30-34	2.272	2.885	2.091	1.545
35-39	4.092	3.571	3.111	2.727
40-44	3.182	4.375	3.75	3.333
45-49	3.308	3.25	3.0	3.231
50-54	3.4	3.333	3.5	-

TABLE 8.7

Proportion of married females according to income category (as a percentage)

Age Group \ Income Group	Less than Rs. 3,000 %	Rs. 3,000 - 7,000 %	Rs.7,000 - 10,000 %	Rs. 10,000 and above %	Sri Lanka %
15 - 19	3.3	3.4	-	-	10.3
20 - 24	32.0	50	22.2	18.2	45.9
25 - 29	80.0	68	44.4	28.6	73.5
30 - 34	86.4	84.6	72.7	63.6	85.9
35 - 39	95.4	100	77.7	100	-

GRAPH 8.1

Age specific mean parity according to income level

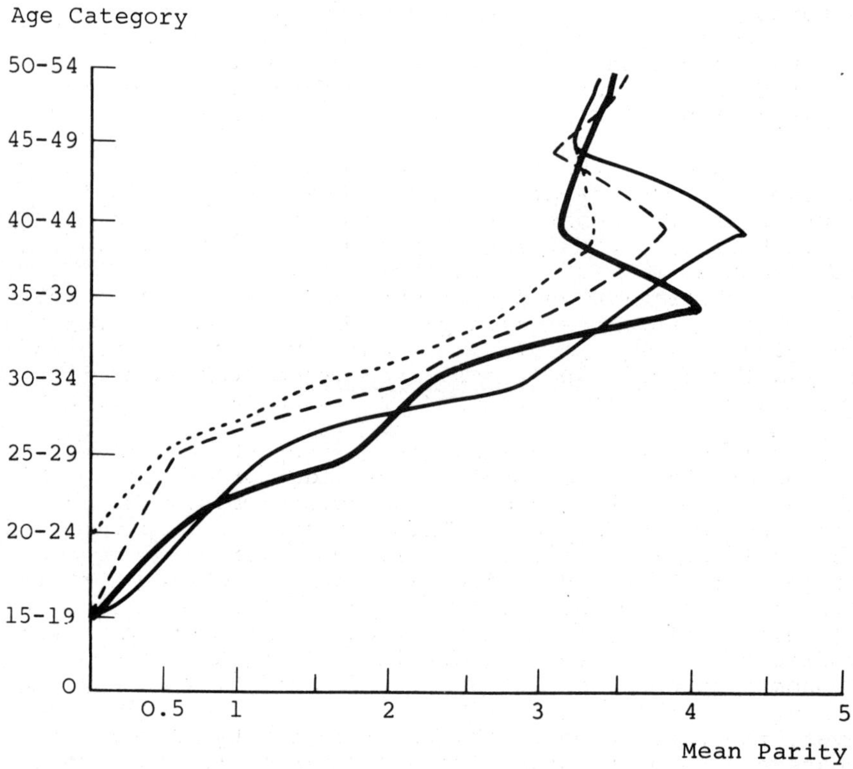

1. ▬▬ = Income below Rs. 3,000/=

2. —— = Income Rs. 3,000-Rs. 7,000/=

3. ---- = Income Rs. 7,000-Rs. 10,000/=

4. ······ = Income Rs. 10,000 & above

Socio-Economic Setting

The framework used in this paper to analyse family size decisions in a rural context stresses the importance of the socio-economic changes that have been going on in Aluthgama-Bogamuwa, as well as in the country as a whole.

When compared with many other parts of Sri Lanka, the Western province where the village is situated has a larger population in the non-agricultural employment sector. Most of the industrial ventures during the last twenty years have been located in the Western province, i.e. nearly 75%, and this has helped to increase the proportion of non-agricultural employment in the area. Therefore the impact of industrialization has reached various parts of Sri Lanka in different degrees.

The basic change in the socio-economic system of Aluthgama-Bogamuwa over the past twenty years has been a change in its employment structure, and the resulting pattern of income levels. The establishment of industries in the locality[2] provided not only employment to some of the villages in the area but it also encouraged a substantial number of outsiders to settle in the village. These changes had both positive and negative effects on the original village population; employment opportunities were created for a few, while sales and fragmentation of land furthered the process of increasing landlessness (see Table 8.3).

Though it is clear that a substantial proportion of landless and small-holders have been employed outside agriculture, the well paid jobs are in the hands of the economically well-off groups or land-owning families. This is mainly a result of wealthier individuals having been able to go for higher education and get into better paid jobs as teachers, office workers and other technical employment. The distribution of income in the village, therefore, is highly skewed. This in turn appears to be reflected in differential fertility among the various socio-economic strata (see Tables 8.3, 8.4 and 8.5).

However, the estimation of the Total Fertility Rate for each income category gives an unrealistic picture of the pattern if based on $\frac{(P3)^2}{P2}$ as compared with $\frac{(P40-49)}{-}$ + 10% (see Table 8.1). This is partly a result of the small size of the sample when the total population is divided into four income categories and partly due to the changing pattern of fertility among the

---

2. For example, the State Hardware Corporation at Yakkala is two miles away, the National Textile Mills at Veyangoda, five miles away and the other at Thulhiriya, 15 miles away from Aluthgama-Bogamuwa. In addition there is a coconut processing mill (medium size) in the village itself.

younger age groups. Therefore if (age specific) Mean Parity is taken as an indicator of fertility it can be seen that fertility declines somewhat with increasing income levels. This is clearly seen among the younger age groups as compared to older age groups where the difference is insignificant, and shows that the fertility decline in the village is a recent trend (see Table 8.6 and Graph 8.1).

Another crude measure that can be used here is the average number of children born to mothers of various income categories. This indicates a declining average except for the third income group.

Income Category Annual Income	Average No. of Children per Mother (aged 15-54)
1. less than Rs. 3,000	3.57
2. Rs. 3,000 - 7,000	3.36
3. Rs. 7,000 - 10,000	3.68
4. Rs. 10,000 and above	3.26

The average number of children per mother in Aluthgama-Bogamuwa is significantly smaller than comparable Indian figures. On the other hand, the disparity between the average number of children per mother for each income category is only marginal. Therefore the recent decline in fertility, as well as the differential fertility among various income groups, has to be explained in terms of other socio-economic variables rather than relating this solely to rising incomes.

In fact the decline in fertility as well as the somewhat differential rates can be largely correlated with two factors: rising age at marriage, and reduction in marital fertility.

The average age at marriage for females in Sri Lanka has been rising from 20.7 in 1946, to 22.1 in 1963 and 23.5 in 1971. In Colombo district it was as high as 24.7 in 1971. Similarly for males it has been rising from 24.6 in 1946 to 28 in 1971 (see Fernando, 1975).

The village data clearly indicate the increasing number of unmarried females in the reproductive age group (15-45). Table 8.7 illustrates the proportion of married females per age group 15-39.

The proportion of married females increases with age, but decreases with increasing income level. In all income groups a substantial proportion of females aged 15-19 are unmarried, and this is partly a result of increasing numbers of the school-going population in this age category. For middle and higher income groups this is more prominent, as many females even in their late teens enter into higher education. For example, the percentage of unmarried females who remain as students in this age category (15-19) increases from 24% for the lowest income group, to 32%, 60% and 100% respectively up to the highest income group.

Nevertheless the high proportion of unmarried females in all social groups highlights certain other factors in a changing social structure, particularly in relation to the institution of marriage. It is basically a question of increasing difficulties in finding suitable marriage partners. Couples marry within a range of socially accepted ages, and postpone marriage within that range because of the inability to satisfy the current norms, such as dowry, property ownership, employment and income. This is particularly important in a society where marriage is arranged and involves fulfillment of at least some of these norms. For middle and higher socio-economic groups, postponement of marriage is mainly a result of being unable to find a suitable partner who would fit into their social category and status. The problem of making satisfactory marriage arrangements for young women is made more difficult by the high degree of female unemployment in Aluthgama-Bogamuwa (see Table 8.8). Nearly 59% of the village unemployed are females, and more than 70% of them have had an education for more than eight years, 15% with G.C.E. and higher qualifications.

Yet the large number of unmarried females need not necessarily be related to the high rate of female unemployment in the area alone, but may also be related to the high rate of general unemployment in the country as a whole. The postponement of marriage by males, due to lack of employment opportunities, automatically restricts the demand for suitable female partners in the marriage market. This high rate of unmarried females in the 1970s in Sri Lanka as a whole has been explained as a result of a 'serious marriage squeeze' (Fernando, 1975) aggravated by the unemployment situation. It is the result of a great imbalance between the proportion of males and females in the marriageable age groups (15-29 for females and 20-34 for males). In 1971 there were only 81.1 males per 100 females in this age category, and this situation will not change for some time. The validity of this argument would be substantial if the proportion remains more or less the same when the assumed age difference between a couple is extended to more than five years. However, the reduction in the proportions marrying in their prime child-bearing years, 20-29, plays an important role in fertility reduction.

The age specific fertility differentials in relation to various income categories as explained by the age specific Mean Parity (Table 8.6) are slightly exaggerated by the fact that there is an increasing proportion of unmarried females in the higher income groups. Therefore when the Mean Parity is calculated in relation to the married females for each income category, the differentials become smaller and less significant (compare Table 8.6 and Table 8.9).

TABLE 8.8

Number of unemployed among unmarried females by income group

Age Group	Income less than Rs. 3,000		Rs. 3,000-7,000		Rs. 7,000-10,000		Rs. 10,000 and above	
	No.	Total	No.	Total	No.	Total	No.	Total
15 - 19	17	29	17	28	6	15	All students	21
20 - 24	11	17	14	16	5	7	6	8
25 - 29	3	12	8	8	4	5	3	4
30 - 34	2	3	3	4	3	3	3	3
Total	54%		75%		60%		33%	

TABLE 8.9

Mean parity for married women

Age Group \ Income Group	Less than Rs. 3,000	Rs. 3,000 - 7,000	Rs. 7,000 - 10,000	Rs. 10,000 and above
15 - 19	1.0	2.029	-	-
20 - 24	1.822	1.188	1.5	-
25 - 29	2.166	1.706	1.252	1.5
30 - 34	2.630	3.410	2.876	2.429
35 - 39	4.288	3.571	4.0	2.727

TABLE 8.10

Mean parity according to level of education of females

Age Group \ Years of Education	Less than 4 years	5-7 years	8-10 years	GCE and above
15 - 19	0.5	-	-	-
20 - 24	0.777	0.571	0.452	0.304
25 - 29	1.8	0.667	1.905	0.5
30 - 34	2.818	2.941	2.156	1.5
35 - 39	4.66	3.125	3.35	2.44
40 - 44	3.18	5.150	2.5	3.33
45 - 49	3.923	3.80	2.09	3.0
50 - 54	2.111	4.11	2.33	-

Factors Affecting Fertility Behaviour

Declining marital fertility poses an enquiry into fertility behaviour patterns. In urban societies, parents tend to think in terms of costs of children and utility derived from them. Economists have been trying to analyse fertility behaviour in relation to utility derived from children, and therefore tend to consider the quantity and quality of children in relation to income, marginal costs and benefits. These concepts cannot be applied to rural societies - in the strictest sense - where people believe in *karma* (fate), and usually say, "If a child has to be born we cannot avoid it, because it is his *karma*". Yet the expected utility may have certain cost considerations in the parents' minds. For example, the following statements are from different types of husbands who belong to the lowest income group:

> "I am satisfied with the two children I have, and do not want to have any more, because I can't afford it."
>
> "I wanted only three or four children, more boys and one or two girls. Since all the children were girls I had to go on until I had a fifth one - a son."
>
> "I wish these rascals were unborn. We didn't know anything about family planning in our days."

The increasing cost of living is reflected not only in the higher cost of children but also affected total family budgets of low income groups. In the early 60s the cost of raising children for the poor was not so great, because the consumer-subsidy scheme and other welfare facilities, such as free health and education, not only reduced the real cost of bringing up younger children, but also benefitted the family. An additional child meant an additional free rice ration card to the family. However, since the recent increase in the cost of food and other items along with a cut in the rice ration (from 4 pounds per week per person to 2 pounds), the low income earners have been compelled to think of their family size.

A few brief case studies collected in Aluthgama-Bogamuwa may help to illustrate some of the motivations in fertility behaviour operating among different socio-economic strata.

Yeunis, a landless labourer of 45 years is married to 34 year old Josepia. Although they belong to the Potter caste, they do not earn much income from their craft, because they have difficulty in securing sufficient raw material which needs to be brought from a distant area at a high price. Josepia produces pots whenever she can, and earns about Rs.200 once every three months by selling them in the local market. Yeunis works as a casual labourer in the nearby brick laying industry, and earns no more than Rs. 175 per month, which hardly suffices to maintain the family.

Yeunis and Josepia have one set of male twins aged seven who both attend school. Due to the rising cost of living they found it increasingly more difficult to buy even the most essential foods for the family and to pay for their children's education. These constraints motivated them to limit the number of their children. They are determined to educate their children so that when they will be grown up they may find better employment and will not have to depend on casual unskilled labour for their livelihood. Though Yeunis has not been contacted by any Family Planning official, his wife had advice after child birth and subsequently had herself sterilised.

Poverty, however, does not always result in fertility control. The relationship between the socio-economic factors and fertility behaviour appears to differ under different conditions. If children help to increase the family income there is no incentive for the parents to limit the number of children they produce.

The case of Sirisena and his wife illustrates this. They moved into Aluthgama-Bogamuwa five years ago and have been employed ever since as manual labourers at the coconut mill. He is 43 years old and his wife is about 35. They have seven children ranging in ages from 15 to 2 years.

Employment in the coconut mill gave them the opportunity to exploit their children's labour and make them contributors to the family income. An individual unskilled labourer can earn no more than Rs. 6 per day. Therefore the more members of a family go out to work the more they can jointly earn. Such unskilled work can readily be performed even by young children.

Sirisena and his family live on the premises of the factory and their household duties are shared by his wife and elder children. Since their children could help in the work done and thereby contribute to the overall family income they were not keen on sending them to school. The eldest daughter had no education whatsoever, while the two sons aged 13 and 11 left school after having completed the fifth form. Only the youngest daughter, who is only seven years, is still at school.

As long as parents are able to provide the basic essentials for their family, children are not regarded as a burden, particularly if children contribute to the family's income from the early age of 10, and also free adult labour by looking after their younger siblings. It seems that parents who themselves had little or no education do not consider investing in their offspring's education, possibly because they are more interested in their children's immediate rather than future earning capacities. In such cases a larger number of children means more income for the family and therefore there is no incentive to reduce fertility.

The attitude of the employed worker is to maintain his standard of living in the face of rising costs. In a system where the extended family is important, it is not only the cost of his own children that he would have to bear, but also that of his parents and younger siblings. Therefore the factory worker or the office worker is forced to think of the number of children as an additional liability in his struggle to maintain his living standard.

The case of Wimal Jayaratne exemplifies this. He is 28 years old and employed as a machine operator at the National Textile Corporation at Veyangoda. His monthly income is about Rs.500, which is the average income of an employed worker in a large scale factory, and also for an office worker.

His parents were very poor and had only half an acre of land; the father did casual work in the area. After he and his elder brother found employment in the textile factory the father stopped working as a casual labourer, and the sons supported their parents.

When Wimal was about twenty five years he married his girl friend from the same village without the approval of her parents, who opposed the marriage because they were better off than Wimal's family, and wanted to give her in marriage to a person of similar social standards. As her parents were against him he had to marry her secretly and, as a result, she was completely cut off from her family and was not given anything as dowry. A few months after the marriage a family dispute over land led his mother to separate from the father, and she came to live in Wimal's house, which she had given to him. The dispute was over half an acre of land, which was given to the eldest son by the father without it being divided among the three sons. She and her youngest son stayed at Wimal's house while the father stayed with the eldest son.

Wimal wanted to maintain a better standard of living compared with his parents. Therefore, he reconstructed the old house, bought new furniture, and various other household equipment. Sometimes he had to work overtime in order to add more to his wages. In addition he borrowed from a relative an acre of paddy land, to work on a tenancy basis. He cultivated this land with the aid of hired labour. Now he has a son about 18 months old, and his wife is expecting another child. After the first child's birth he did not want to have another one, at least for some time. He said "one is more than enough nowadays, especially as my wife doesn't want to have another one in the near future, she has so much to do at home". Even though he did not want to have a second child at least for another two years, his wife conceived unexpectedly, and now he says that "we will not have any more children: It is our fault we did not seek doctor's advice". Even before he married he had decided the number of children they were going to have.

By observation, he realised the disadvantages of having a large family. For example, his own uncle, who has four daughters and a son, finds it difficult to maintain his family, even though he has a job as a driver in one of the government departments. His uncle is really worried about his daughters; it is going to be a great burden for him when the time comes to get them married, as he doesn't have any property or savings to give them as dowry. Even if he can educate them, he wouldn't be able to find them any employment. Wimal was advised by a number of his friends and relatives, who had already had more children, and more problems, not to have any more than two children. Now he intends to seek doctor's advice after the second childbirth.

In a way it is a great help that he has his mother and the younger brother at home. They take care of the child and help his wife in the housework, even though he finds it difficult to provide the necessary comforts for them. Very often his mother goes to her brother and spends a few days there, as she feels she should not be too much of a burden to her son.

The members of the top social stratum appear to be most concerned with maintaining a modern urban life style, while at the same time exercising the role of landlord. Many of them own substantial amounts of land in addition to being employed in well paid jobs. In contrast to the landlords in traditional rural communities, these groups are more enterprising, as well as educated. They invest their surplus income in new business ventures like small-scale confectionary works, textile printing, pottery making (using hired labour), furniture industry, and also in land. On the other hand they spend substantially on household equipment, furniture, vehicles, refrigerators, electric fans and other luxury items. Their family size decisions do not depend on their ability to support children, but on various other factors, such as their attitude towards a better family life with a small number of children, preference for luxury comsumption, their own freedom, and possibly most important, on the prospects of their children's future. The following case study of Sicil Seneviratne illustrates the attitude of the urbanised rural elite.

Sicil is the youngest son of a leading landlord in the Yakkala area, who under British rule was awarded *Muhanfiram vidane* - a status appointment - for his services to the government. After the death of his father he inherited most of his land, while his brothers were well educated and employed in high positions in the ministries as Commissioners. His marriage to one of his cousins (who was a teacher) added more land from the same area, and now he has about 25 acres of high land and about 8 acres of paddy, as well as a house given on rent. He has only two sons aged 19 and 15 years who are attending a well known school in Colombo. He did not want to have any more children as it was not his intention to have a large family; he wanted to educate his sons in one of the best schools and give them all the necessary comforts.

Consequently he removed the children from the village school when they were very young and sent them to a school in Colombo, with the help of his brother, with whom the children are staying now. Even though he can find employment for his eldest son - who has passed the advanced G.C.E. level examination - he wants him to continue his studies in the engineering faculty at the University. He is keen to invest more in his children's education and is trying his best to push them up the social ladder of success.

These case studies of families belonging to diverse social strata all indicate the importance of education as a variable affecting fertility decisions.

The overall decline in fertility over the past few years can certainly be related to the general improvement in education and health facilities in the area. Free education has provided many villagers with sufficient knowledge to understand the advice given under the family planning programme through public health services. Mothers are advised by doctors at hospitals and are frequently visited by the public health midwives.

Levels of education among females correspond fairly well with their fertility patterns. The percentage distribution of Aluthgama Bogamuwa females according to the number of years of education is as follows[4]:

Less than 4 years of education	=	22.5
5 - 7 years of education	=	23.9
8 -10 years of education	=	33.5
G.C.E. and higher education	=	20.1

Most of the higher income group females have received a longer period of education than those in low income groups, and this is closely related to their fertility pattern. This correlation between level of education and fertility can be seen especially among the younger age groups (below 39 years), compared with the older age groups where there is no such regular pattern (see Table 8.10, and also Graph 8.2).

Conclusion

In this paper I outlined the demographic changes which I observed in Aluthgama-Bogamuwa. I showed that there are clear signs of a demographic transition and attempted to relate the declining population growth rate to socio-economic differences. Though the various socio-economic and educational strata display similar fertility behaviour, it is important to distinguish the different motivations operative for each of them. Educational facilities, as well as the availability of maternity care and advice, have provided the necessary background for a fairly successful programme of family planning.

---

4. The majority of the educated come from the younger age groups.

Among the poorest, the conscious awareness of the costs of a large number of children have convinced them of the need to limit family size. This is particularly the case among the younger age groups with a few years of education, as illustrated in Yeunis's case. Among these groups termination of fertility is a common feature. By contrast Sirisena's case shows that lack of education and the availability of child labour make for high fertility.

For the families of the middle stratum, with an annual income between Rs. 3,000-10,000, the problem of poverty is less important in influencing their fertility decisions than their concern with maintaining and improving their standard of living, in the knowledge that additional children involve additional costs. For them children represent a considerable expense, particularly because of the high rate of unemployment, which may mean that their offspring remain dependents until they reach their twenties or even thirties. They represent the stratum which is most concerned with upward mobility, although many of its members belong to extended families and therefore carry larger financial burdens.

Wimal's case exemplifies the newly emerging meritocracy in Sri Lanka, who are determined to secure a better future for their children, but who carry extended family commitments which weigh like a millstone round their necks.

Parents of the upper stratum on the other hand, are concerned about the quality of their children, and therefore limit family size and invest substantially in their education. Like Sicil, many other rich parents educate their children in the well known schools in Colombo, and are interested in improving their socio-economic standards through higher education. Spacing, as well as limiting the number of children to their own ideal size, is common among this upper stratum.

The different motivations I discussed which operate among the different socio-economic categories bear important theoretical as well as practical implications. In the theoretical sphere my findings indicate that different household decision-making models are necessary for each social category, and one would hope that planners are able to draw important lessons from the account presented here.

GRAPH 8.2

Age specific mean parity according to education level

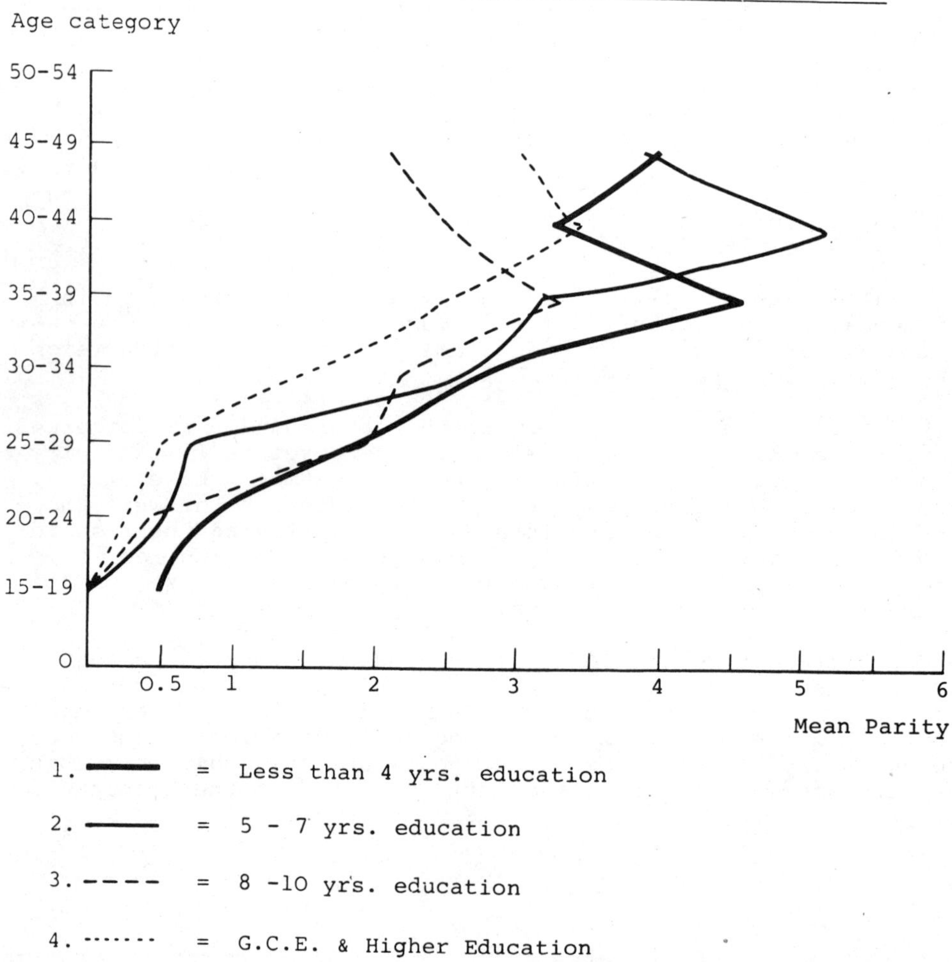

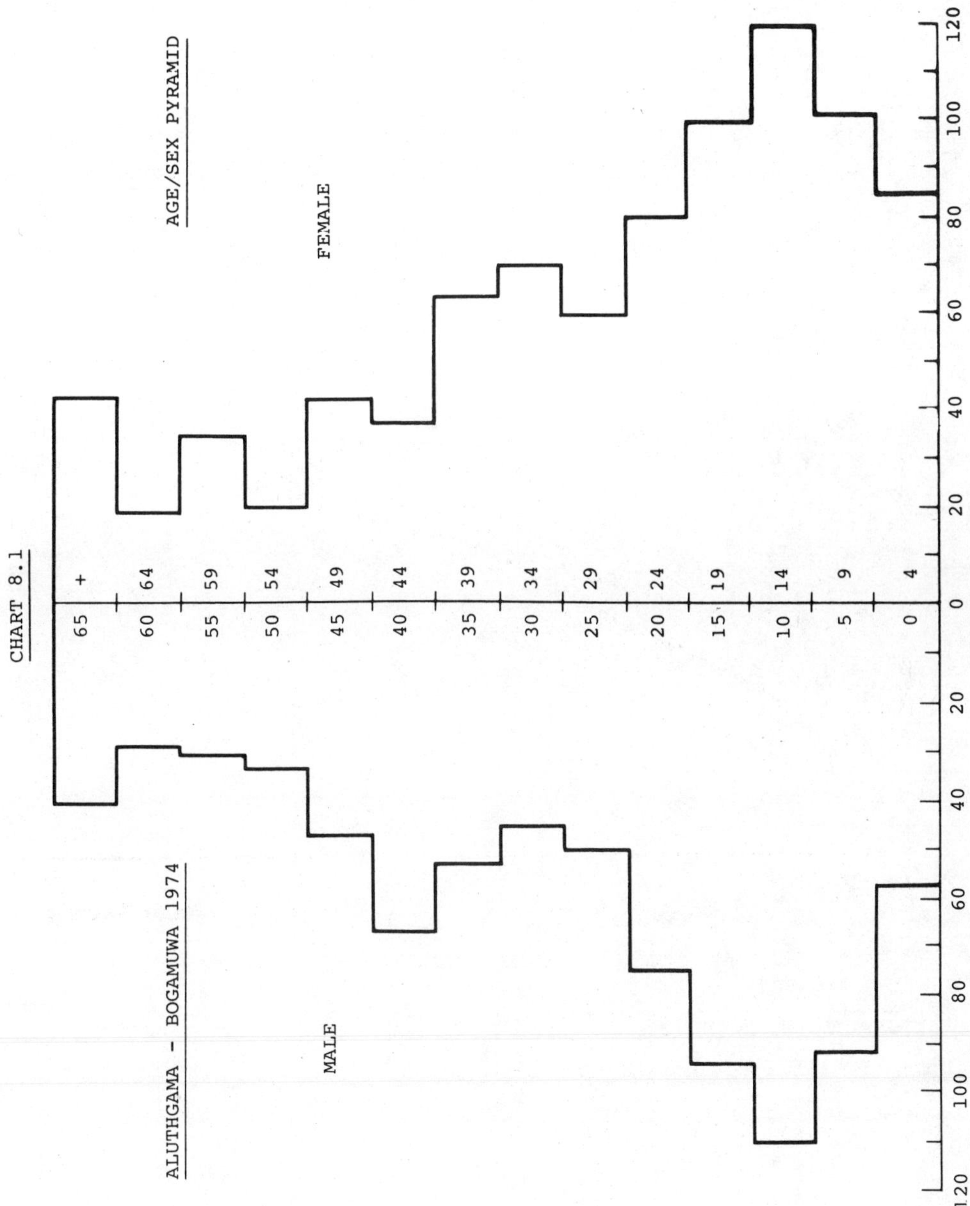
CHART 8.1
ALUTHGAMA - BOGAMUWA 1974
AGE/SEX PYRAMID
MALE
FEMALE
65 +
60 64
55 59
50 54
45 49
40 44
35 39
30 34
25 29
20 24
15 19
10 14
5 9
0 4
120 100 80 60 40 20 0 20 40 60 80 100 120

CHAPTER 9

EDUCATION, POVERTY AND FERTILITY AMONG THE WATAITA OF KENYA

INTRODUCTION

In this paper I discuss the relationship between education, poverty and fertility based on twelve months fieldwork amongst the Wataita tribe of Southern Kenya.

Given the present stage of economic development in rural Taita, the household as a socio-economic unit is distinctive more for its consumption than its production activities. Factors such as land consolidation and the accompanying individualisation of land ownership rights have contributed to a situation whereby the role of the agrarian based household as a self-sufficient socio-economic unit has been considerably restricted. An additional factor is the productive capacity of the land, which is not sufficient to feed the population for the whole year. Unlike the low-lying plains, the hill areas receive adequate rainfall, but the productivity of the hill lands is limited by the topography, which represents a prohibitive factor for the introduction of mechanized agriculture. Agriculture, which is characterized by *shamba*[1] work, is therefore a labour intensive activity done largely by women and children.

As a result of these factors the household is often able to produce only six months food supply, and sometimes less. Household survival for the next six months depends on its earning capacity outside agriculture, so members have to participate in the wider economy in order to increase their income and to enable them to buy necessities. These two aspects of the household economy should be seen as complementary, as opposed to the notion of a 'dual economy'.

Non-agricultural economic activities open to household members may be classified into three groups, namely (in descending order of remuneration), salary earning, self-employment and casual labouring.

Salary earners would include District and County Council Administrators at all levels, as well as members of the professions, such as teachers, police, bank clerks, medical staff, technicians etc. Also subordinate staff, such as secretaries, telephonists, groundsmen and office messengers.

1. A *shamba* is a small farm.

The self-employed category includes tailors, artisans, radio/watch repairers, carpenters, masons, hawkers, shopkeepers, hoteliers, bus and lorry owners and *matatu*[2] operators. This self-employed group play many different roles - a businessman owning a shop is often also an artisan, a builder and at times, a farmer.

The casual labourers constitute the rural unemployed and under-employed. These may be male labourers who seek any work available for a meagre income. They may scoop sand for brick-making from the river-beds, till somebody's farm, carry luggage or perform any other casual job available. Female workers are usually barmaids (who generally double as prostitutes), extra-hand farm workers and house-maids. Boys between 6-14 years old could also be included in this category. They are usually school children who have to take on casual work after school hours or during the holidays in order to contribute to the family's income. Included in this category are those who have finished their 4 years of free primary education and are unable to pay the school fees to continue their education. These working children come noticeably from poorer families and mostly have widowed mothers.

A household's self-sufficiency vis-a-vis its socio-economic status therefore depends on two sets of interrelated criteria.

Firstly it must have a sufficient supply of labour for its agricultural production. The main source of this labour is the immediate household unit. A random sample of 36 households (9.5% of the total households in my universe) with a total number of 105 adults, gave the following results. About 36% did not engage in agricultural work. These were mostly men, although there were a few business women included. 46% were engaged in agricultural work. This included mostly women, their grown-up children and some men. Of the total labour force engaged in agriculture, only 1.9% were hired labourers.

Secondly, the household must have some possibility of earning a steady income from some (or all) of its household population through permanent non-agricultural employment. Since high income-earning capacity is directly related to a level of academic achievement, investment in education is the only course open to a household unit.

---

2. *Matatu* is a term once used to refer to taxis which had no licence from the Transport Licensing Board and hence operated illegally. A Presidential pronouncement has removed this obstacle, thus allowing any owner of a car or small pick-up van to turn his vehicle into a taxi.

Education and Income as Determinants of Fertility

Education provides the essential means of access to the necessary non-agricultural income among Wataita families. Though education is in theory free for the levels below 4 and above 12 years of training, in practice there are considerable expenses involved for parents schooling children of all ages.

The higher the education of the individual, the greater appears to be her/his concern with the cost of educating children. This is reflected in Table 9.1, which shows an inverse correlation between the educational levels of the 62 respondents in the sample on the one hand and the average number of children each desires.

TABLE 9.1

Educational Level and Desired Number of Children

Household head's education by years	No. of respondents	Average children desired
No education	18	7.6
1 - 4	12	7.0
5 - 8	21	7.1
9 -12	8	4.6
13 -14	3	4.0

Since the level of educational achievement is highly linked with the level of income, parents usually attempt to educate all of their children. A household finding it hard to fulfill this function may employ one or a combination of the following strategies. One possibility would be to sacrifice a daughter's education, if the family was faced with the problem of choosing whom to educate. This is in keeping with the norm that the male children are regarded as a better asset than female children. Alternatively the household could terminate the education of the eldest, forcing him to earn a steady income so that he could contribute to educating his younger siblings. Finally the household could sell or mortgage some of its property. In this case land is the easiest marketable commodity for which to find a buyer.

It can be deduced, therefore, that in their endeavours to have at least one successful son, the poorer strata is inexorably driving itself into landlessness. This could be either directly through the outright sale of land in order to finance children's education, or through the inheritance system, which stipulates that sons have to be given equal shares of their father's land. This involves further fragmentation of the existing small land-holdings, so that, within a generation or two, land-holdings will be unviable by virtue of their small size. Consequently, the poorest will be forced to sell their land. The rich, by amalgamating many such small holdings, could then use the land for cash cropping by employing cheap labour which is abundant in rural areas, or rent it out either for farming or building permanent residential houses. This process has already happened in Maragoli, Western Keyna, as shown by Joseph Ssennyonga in his concept of the 'elite roadside ecology' (see p. 62).

A random sample study of 36 Wataita households indicates a direct correlation between income and education on the one hand, and an inverse correlation between these two variables and the average number of children per household on the other.

Table 9.2 indicates that the dividing line between those households with less than £60 per capita annual income and those earning more appears to be particularly important. Below this strategic level households have an average of 5.4 children and their head has an average number of four years formal education. The respective figures for the higher income categories are 3.6 children and six years formal education.

The relationship between poorer households and their large numbers of children may be accounted for by the fact that they find themselves in a vicious circle of low income and low education, where large numbers of children represent the only hope of making a break-through. It is precisely within this predicament of scarcity of land, lack of employment opportunities and low levels of education, that the poor perceive their solution in terms of larger numbers of children. They assume that more children increase their chances of at least one or two of their offspring being able to break the poverty-generating cycle. More often than not, however, this breakthrough does not occur and the large numbers of children cause the poor to continue to move along the downward spiral of poverty. Only *post facto* - after a poor family has had many children without achieving the hoped for break-through - does the parental generation begin to express the view that they would have done better with fewer children. However, the occasional success story, when one child of a poor family becomes its saviour, continues to encourage the poorest families to have larger numbers of children. This attitude can be compared with the gambling phenomenon: the majority of people prefer a smaller chance of a greater reward to a greater chance of a smaller reward.

TABLE 9.2

Income, Education and Numbers of Dependent Children

Annual per capita income (£ sterling)*	Household Heads No.	Household Heads %	Combined percentages	Average No. of dependent children per house hold head+		Household head average years of formal education	Combined averages (years)
Below 20	7	19	66	6.4	5.4	3.0	4.0
20 - 39	6	17		6.5		4.5	
40 - 59	11	30		4.6		4.4	
60 - 79	7	19	34	4.1	3.6	4.0	6.0
80 - 99	3	9		2.0		5.5	
100 -200	2	6		4.5		9.0	

* The income categories in this column are based on those used in Table 25 of the ILO Employment Mission Kenya Report.

\+ There is an even age distribution of household heads within the different income categories. Therefore, the difference in the average number of dependent children between households below and above an annual per capita income of £60 cannot be accounted for by difference in domestic life cycle phases.

Concern about Family Size

The 62 sample respondents were asked to give reasons for their desired number of children and their sex composition. Their answers fall into two categories:

Economic considerations

Exactly half cited economic-oriented reasons, while the rest were primarily motivated by social variables. The former expressed concern about the scarcity of land and the lack of employment opportunities. 75 per cent of the respondents perceived this in terms of the cost involved in bringing up large numbers of children. More than half of these respondents were mainly worried about the difficulty of earning the necessary money to raise children. Statements like 'My means of raising children are limited' or 'My husband is not permanently employed' or 'The cost of living is high; although I am fond of children I cannot afford to have as many as I would like', reflect this. Others appeared primarily worried about the scarcity of land and said e.g. 'Our plot is too small for more than two sons'.

The strength of the economic pressures facing the society can be illustrated by three infanticide cases (one attempted and two successful) by three unmarried mothers. In the attempted case, the mother threw the infant into a pit latrine and tried to drown the child by using a long pole. Miraculously, the child was rescued. In the other two cases the infants were abandoned in the bush and were discovered dead the following morning.

In each case the mothers were unmarried and came from the category with less than £20 p.a. per capita income. Within this category 20% of all male children born alive are automatically landless because their mothers are unmarried and, being women, customary law prohibits them from inheriting land from their fathers. In fact the motive given by all three mothers for their actions was the fear of watching their children (all males) growing up into a landless group.

Social considerations

As mentioned above 50 per cent of the sample respondents were primarily concerned with social considerations in their attitudes to the family size and sex composition of their children.

About half of this category indicated a preference for having more male than female children, because 'boys will stay with the house - they provide stability and continuity', or 'boys are strength in the world; girls move to other places'. The importance of old age security as a consideration in deciding on the number of children per couple emerged clearly when most of these informants said that they expected their families to take care of them in the event of their illness. They went on to stress that they hoped their children would look after them when they themselves were too old to work.

Some have a fatalistic approach, indicating a felt lack of choice in the matter by saying 'Whoever and however many children are born, each has a destiny'. A few gave traditional reasons for having many children, again with a bias towards male children: 'I want so many children because our ancestors did not use birth control', or 'My own father had more than a dozen kids - if he managed to raise them, so I should be able to raise mine'. Child-bearing as the traditional function of women was mentioned by some respondents, who suggested that it was unnecessary to limit numbers of children because 'It is a woman's duty to produce - not all of them will be clever - but I want to be helped when I am old'.

Status considerations motivate others to have many children. One man, for instance said that he regards children as prestigious. 'I want to look like an Indian Sultan, surrounded by my large family'. Yet others took into account the possibility of heavy child mortality and desired a specific number of children. 'If three die I want to be left with at least three'. Again, others seem more aware of the transitory stage their community finds itself in and they tend to be more pragmatic as to whether or not to have more male than female children: 'Girls help parents more. But boys like eating alone with their wives; daughter-in-laws ignore their mother-in-laws; although boys mean stability'.

A few respondents mentioned the basic satisfaction derived from child-bearing and would not like to limit their numbers of children because 'one feels worthwhile with children'.

These various considerations may help to throw light on the fact that despite economic pressures, parents still go for many children, such that the annual rate of population growth in Kenya is between 3.6 - 3.9 per cent (1973 Demographic Baseline Survey Report, Central Bureau of Statistics, Kenya Ministry of Finance and Planning).

Conclusion

This essay attempted to highlight the interlinkages between education, poverty and rapid population growth. There are, of course, other important influences affecting fertility patterns which have not been included in this analysis, although they do contribute to this social phenomenon. Ethnicity is one such variable, which operates both at macro and micro-level; religion is another. Both of these have been left out because they lack the direct causal relationship which exists between education, income and fertility.

The three-dimensional relationship with its mutual reinforcement has to be broken down before rural communities can be expected to respond positively to both government and private organisation programmes aiming at fertility reductions.

Intermediate technologies should be provided to make hill agriculture less laborious. Moreover, the water that goes unused down the valleys should be piped up to the hill tops for human consumption and irrigation. This would help to put more land under cultivation and enable farmers to go in for multi-cropping.

The officials responsible for publicising contraceptives should be young people of both sexes, instead of as now, old women beyond their menopause, who are in no position to practise what they preach. Altogether, family planning publicity could be made more effective by integrating it into the overall strategy for rural development.

Perhaps what is needed is a communal approach towards the whole problem of rapid population growth and poverty. This approach envisages the communalization of the decision of having children in relation to the communal resources available, as for instance in China - see Chapter 11. This implies a shift of emphasis from attempts to attain low fertility at the household level - which ignores the possibility that the community may remain poor - to a positive stress on a prosperous community, which may then be able to support a high aggregate level of fertility. If the basic emphasis was on the community and not on the individual, then perhaps the poverty syndrome might be eradicated.

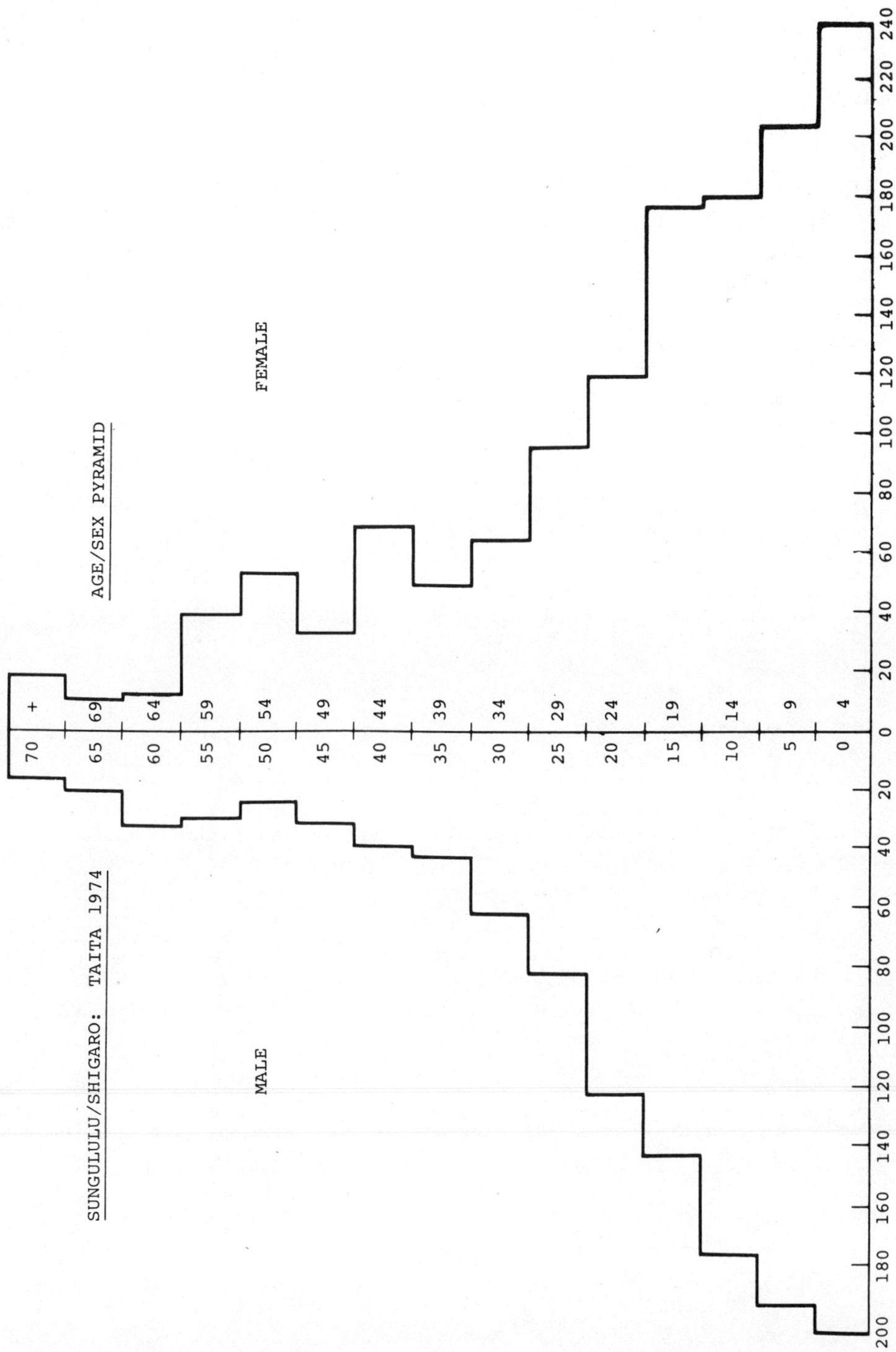
SUNGULULU/SHIGARO: TAITA 1974
AGE/SEX PYRAMID
MALE
FEMALE
70 +
65 69
60 64
55 59
50 54
45 49
40 44
35 39
30 34
25 29
20 24
15 19
10 14
5 9
0 4
200 180 160 140 120 100 80 60 40 20 0 20 40 60 80 100 120 140 160 180 200 220 240

CHART 9.1

CHAPTER 10

CHANGING PRODUCTION RELATIONS AND POPULATION GROWTH

INTRODUCTION

In this paper I attempt to explain the pattern of population growth in a North Indian village in relation to changes in production conditions since the late nineteenth century. This village was first studied in 1925-26 (Asthana, 1929). No detailed quantitative data is available for the period between 1925 and 1974, and therefore the changing historical conditions during this period have been largely constructed on the basis of information received from the villagers during my field visit in 1974-75.

I focus here on the change in production relations since the introduction of the 'new agricultural technology' and its impact on attitudes towards family size. I argue that new technologies and higher productivity have led to a decline in the extent of sharecropping and an increase in the inequalities. Small peasants are being forced to lease out their small plots of land because of non-ownership of the basic means of production, for example, a pair of bullocks. Also, more and more of the poor villagers are being pushed out to look for sources of income outside the village's agricultural economy. Consequently, because of these changing relationships, couples no longer need a large number of children. Yet it seems that fertility is unlikely to decline until the mortality rates - particularly of infant mortality - are brought down.

Ramdaua is the fictitious name of the village which I studied. An earlier study (Asthana, 1929) gives the correct name of the village, although individual hamlets are not mentioned, since at that time records were only available at the 'revenue village'[1] level. Ramdaua is the central hamlet or village of a cluster of ten which together comprise a revenue village. It is located in tehsil Sandila, which is in District Hardoi of central Uttar Pradesh. In 1925-26, the revenue village as a whole was studied, but in 1974-75, I concentrated only on the village Ramdaua.

---

1. A revenue village is the smallest administrative unit in rural India. These units were created in the British period for the purposes of evaluation and collection of revenue. Thus a revenue village can consist of one or more residential clusters each called a hamlet in the official language. But, locally, people refer to these residential clusters or hamlets as *Gaon*. Generally, the revenue unit has a main 'village' which is surrounded by smaller 'villages' and the revenue village is named after the main village.

The pre-1925 *Taluqdari*[2] Period

High Mortality

In 1925, the revenue village had a population of 1,525 and a total area, agricultural and residential, of 2,272 acres. Thus the total land-man ratio was 1.490 acres per person. On the basis of the cultivated area (including seasonal fallow) of 1,172 acres that year, the land-man ratio was 0.772 acre per person. However, the distribution of rights to land was extremely unequal and some had no access at all. The earlier study gives the following distribution of the population (including all family members) according to 'agricultural class':

Proprietor	1
Cultivators	1,205
Farm labourers	275
Landless labourers	144
Total	1,625[3]

The *taluqdar* was the only proprietor. He had 118 acres for his own cultivation, out of which 58 acres were cultivated, probably with farm labourers and wage labourers, and 60 acres which were cultivated by 20 tenants-at-will. Almost every family in the village had to provide a certain amount of free labour during the year for the *taluqdar*. Prior to 1920, a large proportion of the tenancies were of occupancy type but the tenants lacked legal status. As a result of an armed rebellion, by 1924

2. A *taluqdar* was a king (*raja*) of a *taluqa* or estate. A *taluqa* could vary from a few hundred acres to hundreds of thousands of acres. In District Hardoi, in 1926, about 450 villages were *taluqdari*, belonging to 20 estates; 1,569 villages were not *taluqdari*. The *taluqdar* of Ramdaua ruled over 15 villages including ten belonging to the 'revenue village' Ramdaua. He was responsible for the revenue of these fifteen villages. The *taluqdar* was the sole proprietor who had the right to collect agricultural tax from the tenants cultivating the rest of the land; part of this tax was given to the government as land revenue.

3. In this table, taken from the earlier study, the number of villagers total 1,625, whereas it was in fact 1,525. Despite this inexplicable error the general pattern remains clear.

TABLE 10.1

Village land distribution, 1925 and 1975

Land distribution (1925)

Land cultivated	Tenants Number	Tenants %	
0 - 6.5 kb*	78	27.9)	43
6.5 - 12 kb	43	15.4)	
12 - 21 kb	71	25.4	
21 - 45 kb	70	25.0)	31
45+ kb	17	6.0)	

Source: Asthana, 1929.

Land distribution (1975)

Land-owned	Households Number	Households %	
Landless	25	11.1	
Less than 5 kb*	96	42.6)	63
5+ - 10 kb	46	20.4)	
10+ - 20 kb	42	18.6	
20+ - 50 kb	14	6.2)	7
50+ kb	2	0.88)	

* kb (*Kaccha Bigha*) is the local unit for area measurement. In the earlier (1925) study, 5 kb were taken to be equal to an acre. Actually, 4.8 kb make an acre. (Bigha is the unit used in official records: 3 kb = 1 Bigha and 1.6 Bigha = 1 acre). For comparison, all the land has been converted into kb units.

there were 84% tenancies with full occupancy rights.[4] 6% were non-occupancy tenants, i.e. cultivators. Land distribution figures are given in Table 10.1.

In 1925 31% of the tenants cultivated 21kb or more (4.375 acres or over) and 43.3% cultivated less than 12kb (2.5 acres). Also, the top 16.8% of the tenants cultivated 51% of the cultivated land and the bottom 83.2% cultivated 49%. All the holdings were divided into numerous small scattered plots. The average number of plots per holding was 9. One particular 75kb holding was divided into 27 scattered plots. Therefore permanent improvement of the land was almost impossible. Irrigation was done by 27 wells, only half of which were *pucca* (brick) wells, 57 tanks and a canal. The techniques of irrigation were extremely slow and labour-intensive, as the following description[5] of the three main systems indicates:

> *Beri* or Life system. 'In this system there are four men in two pairs engaged at one place, each pair replacing the other at suitable intervals. They hoist up water from a low level by means of a rectangular basket or *beri* to which two ropes are attached on each of the two small sides, which are held by the two men standing on both sides of the place from which water is to be lifted.'
> *Pur* or *Garra* system. 'The *pur* or *charsa* is a leather bucket for drawing water from the wells. The *pur* is attached to a thick rope or *bariat* which is drawn over a wooden pulley either by 2 or 4 bullocks or 8 or 16 men yoked in pairs. In order to reduce labour there is a regular slope, adjacent to the wells down which the *garra* is drawn.'
> *Dhekuli* or Lever lift. 'The whole mechanism consists of one long beam supported on one or two strong poles at a convenient point. At one end of the beam which is nearer the ground a heavy weight of mud is attached, while at the other a water bucket is hung by means of a long rope sufficient to reach the water level of the well. A man stands at the mount of the well, and when the bucket is full of water, leaves it to come up on account of the weight at the other end of the beam'.

---

4. The high percentage of 'occupancy-type' tenants (relatively high security of tenure) was a result of an armed peasant uprising, described in the earlier study: "The growing discontent among the poorer tenants led to a dangerous outburst in 1922, known as the EKA movement. About 1,200 peasants of this village and ten neighbouring villages came under the spell of an Indian Jack Cade. They attacked the house of the *taluqdar* and the *patwari* and wanted to wrest from them leaseholds (*pattas*) for life. The revolt was suppressed by the sepoys of the estate ... the new Oudh Rent Act brought statutory rights to them and has partly satisfied the most disturbing elements of the village" (Asthana, 1929:21).
5. See Asthana, 1929:56.

As a result of these laborious processes 85.7% of the cultivated area remained un-irrigated, and the intensity of water which was supplied to the irrigated area was very low. Consequently, productivity was also low - particularly when the rains failed.

To make things more difficult for tenants the rent demanded by the *taluqdar* from them was very high. The earlier study found that the 'recorded' rents amounted to 11 - 12% of the net profits from cultivation (output minus cost), whereas the *actual* rents were 20 - 25%. During my field visit in 1974-75, people in the village complained about the old *taluqdari* days when they had to pay heavy rents. Very little food was left for consumption, so that they had to miss their meals quite frequently. Those who complained were mostly 'middle' peasants, who now own from two to four acres. Sub-letting was on the increase in those days, in which case the rent paid by the actual cultivator was even higher. Apart from the rent, the *taluqdari* received gifts and taxes in various forms from each household. Thus, there existed considerable poverty and starvation. The houses of the poorest were mere temporary shelters with no doors or windows. Epidemics and famines were frequent, and consequently mortality rates were very high. This can be shown by examining the revenue village population figures from 1891 - 1921 (Asthana 1929:6).

Total population for revenue village Ramdaua (1891-1921).

Year	Population	Percent change
1891	1,451	
1901	1,307	- 9.9
1911	1,273	- 2.6
1921	1,466	+15.1

Thus the revenue village population increased by only one per cent during the thirty years 1891-1921. This pattern might have been the result, though only partly, of out-migration, but I found no evidence for this explanation in the earlier study. Those were the times of extremely high mortality: unhygienic living conditions, lack of medical facilities and extreme poverty were the main causes. "About 90 per cent of the children up to the age of sixteen years were victims, and at least 40 per cent of the total number of children attacked died. The general rate of mortality for the whole village has gone up from 12 per cent to 15 per cent during the last two years. (Asthana, 1929:10).

The poverty was the result of shortage of land, its skewed distribution, the fragmentation of holdings into small plots and inefficient techniques of production. Consequently, there was low productivity coupled with high rents. Whatever little surplus was generated by the few well-off families was saved for expenditure on social ceremonies associated with birth, death and marriage. The *taluqdar* spent a lot of money on conspicuous consumption: riding elephants, hunting, organising dance and drama and maintaining a large number of domestic servants. Part of the village produce was appropriated as land revenue by the colonial regime. Thus the surplus produced was hardly ever ploughed back into productive investment and the majority of the population was heavily indebted, many of them to the *taluqdar*. Under this form of production organisation and in these living conditions, the village population were faced with the struggle for mere survival; family size became a secondary problem.

The *Taluqdari* Period: 1925-1952: Importance of Subsistence Labour and Sub-letting

In 1925, the revenue village had 512.5 acres of *usar* or barren land and 298.75 acres of forest or bush. Since then most of the forest and bush land has been cleared for cultivation, although deforestation also makes the land *usar* (Whitcombe, 1972). At the same time, some of the *usar* land has been slowly converted into cultivable land by intensive irrigation and manuring, although productivity on such land is quite low and increases very slowly. Between 1925 and 1952, there was also a slight improvement in irrigation techniques. The major change in this respect was the introduction of the Persian wheel.

During the same period, quite a few men from the village used to go out for construction jobs on roads and railways, sometimes three hundred miles away, for periods of a few months. Apart from being a source of income, the building of roads and railways also meant an improvement in the transport system, which facilitated the movement of foodgrains during the times of famine. Due to these factors and a slight increase in productivity in the area under cultivation, some improvements in living conditions occurred. Mortality declined and the village population started increasing steadily. This can be seen from the genealogies of all the village households; a greater proportion of the siblings during this period lived to get married and have children than in previous generations.

The reduction in mortality implies an increase in family size, assuming that fertility is not reduced. Now it is a well known fact that methods of fertility control were not unknown in 'traditional' societies (see e.g. Devereux, (1955); Mandelbaum, (1973); Nag, (1962). In village Ramdaua, abortion by traditional medicines has been known for years and is still practised. Also, I found that the concept of 'spacing' of births (to prevent malnutrition of the mother and the child) has existed for a long time. Therefore the question arises: if the methods were known, why were they not used to limit family size? My hypothesis is that the people of Ramdaua wanted large families, and especially sons. In what follows I attempt to explain this need for a large number of sons in a family.

Even in 1925, it was seen that sub-letting existed and was slowly on the increase. But apart from family labour, farm labour

TABLE 10.2

Consolidated table showing the costs and profits of cultivation per acre cultivated in village Ramdaua 1925/6

Reference to the family budgets studied in the chapters on 'Standard of Living'	No. of members in each family	No. of ploughs in each family	No. of bullocks in each family	Area cultivated by each family	Costs of cultivation: Regular farm labour	Weeding	Irrigation	Reaping and picking	Communal dues	Seed	Cattle and instruments of production	Rent: Amount	Rent: Percentage to net profit	Total costs of cultivation	Cost of cultivation per acre	Total gross profits of cultivation	Total net profits of cultivation	Net profits of cultivation per acre
				Acs.	Rs.	Rs.	Rs.	Rs.	Rs.	Rs.	Rs.	Rs.	Rs.	Rs.	Rs.	Rs.	Rs.	Rs.
1	7	3	6	20	180	50	75	25	30	100	50	200	20	710	35/8	1,665	955	47/12
2	14	2	3	8.5		20	10	10	25	50	10	75	24	200	23/8	515	315	37/1
3	6	2	4	5.2		10	5	5	5	12		33	12	70	13/6	358	288	55/6
4	4			0.6		3	2	1	2	6		8	4	22	36/10	87	65	108/5
5	6	1	2	2.0		8	2/8	2	5	16		8/8	125	42	21	241	199	99/8
6	3			0.3						0/4		1/12		2	6/10	3/8	1/8	4/8

Source: Asthana, (1929:62)

and wage labour[6] were the dominant types of help used for cultivation of the larger holdings. The earlier study analysed the costs and profits of cultivation for six sample households from three economic strata,(see Table 10.2) and shows that in 1925 the costs were a much higher propertion of gross earnings for larger holdings of land and productivity was much lower. Under these conditions of agricultural production, it was rational for tenants with large holdings to sub-let their land, either to tenants with small holdings or to the landless labourers, who had a large supply of family labour. It can be seen from Table 10.2 that family labour is much more productive than either farm or wage labour. Thus a small family with inadequate subsistence labour would find it profitable to sub-let land, even with only a medium-sized land-holding. Again, a greater number of adult males in the family were an advantage in helping to clear more forest-bush land for cultivation.

These production conditions suggest that, despite very unequal rights in land, the distribution of land cultivated changed in favour of families with a large supply of (preferably male) labour. It should be noted here that the higher castes, forming a very small percentage of the population never cultivated their land with family labour, irrespective of household size. For the majority of the population, there was an incentive to have a large family. Consequently, no decline in fertility could be expected; the population increased steadily during 1925-1952.

1952-69: Post *Zamindari* Abolition Period Preparation for Change

As already mentioned, the *taluqdar* was the sole intermediary between the villager and the State for revenue collection. The system of using intermediaries rather than government-appointed revenue collectors was part of a wider administrative system known as *zamindari*. *Zamindari* was abolished in Uttar Pradesh in 1952. Most of the tenants became owners and revenue was paid directly to the State. Official rates were lower than those paid to the *taluqdar*. Basically, however, the distribution of rights over land did not change much. Land holdings continued to be scattered. Techniques of cultivation remained the same and productivity continued to be low. All the large landholdings were given out to a number of sharecroppers, and in that relationship the owner contributed nothing towards the cost of the inputs and appropriated half the produce. A large family thus meant that more land could be leased in for sharecropping, provided the sharecropper owned the basic means of production such as a plough and a pair of bullocks. There were a few families with a large supply of family labour in the village who

6. Farm labour is distinguished from wage labour by the period of employment. In the former case labourers were employed by the major landowners for periods ranging from 6 - 18 months. Wage labour was hired on a casual, daily basis.

leased in a lot of land and have slowly been able to buy more. The land they cultivated showed higher productivity and owners of land are happy to lease out land to such large families. Thus control of fertility would then have made no sense for the majority of the villagers.

The ideology of the large family continued to be rational at the individual level. But the village population was growing and no more land was available for cultivation, given the techniques of production. This implied more fragmentation and an increase in the number of smaller, uneconomic holdings. Land, being private property since 1952, could be sold on the market. An insufficient food supply for a family meant borrowing, which in turn implied mortgaging land, and finally, after continued debt for years, selling it. This process has been continuously taking place in village Ramdaua since 1952. It is in line with what Bailey demonstrated for an Orissa village (1957:61). The population pressure on land and its consequences led to a sharp increase in seasonal migration, especially to the cities of Kanpur and Lucknow. Some young men migrated to Delhi and Bombay. Most of these migrants belong to small and middle peasant families, i.e. owner-cultivators.

Around 1965, a milk co-operative was started in the village and government loans were distributed for buying cows and buffaloes. The sale of milk and its products became an important source of income for the middle peasants, who could afford to buy these cattle. Government loans were given against property owned, mainly land. After *zamindari* abolition in 1952, a land ceiling came into force although it affected only the *taluqdar* family in the village. They had to sell about half of their land and now they have a total of 62 acres.

Land in village Ramdaua was consolidated in 1961-62. The advantages of consolidation fell mainly to those with large land-holdings. For instance, the largest two land-holdings in the village had their land consolidated in plots of ten to twenty acres, whereas a small land-holding of one acre was divided into three or four plots dispersed at distances of up to one mile. Land-consolidation was a necessary condition for any technological improvements in agricultural techniques. Subsequently, electricity was brought to the village in 1969, essentially for irrigation. Government loans, backed by land securities, were available for the purchase of tubewells. All the material conditions were now present for a major change in agricultural production.

1969-1975: Technological Changes

In 1974-75 the village Ramdaua had a cultivated area (including seasonal fallow) of 380 acres, with a population of 1,170. This gives a land-man ratio of 0.324 acre per person, against 0.772 for the revenue village in 1925. On top of this, the distribution of land has become much worse (see Table 10.1). 7% of

TABLE 10.3

Tubewell owners in Ramdaua (1975)

Sample number	No. of tubewells	Land owned (kb.)	Caste	Other occupations
1	3	300	Thakur	One brother working in Lucknow with Fertiliser Corporation of India
2	1	65	Kayastha	Postmaster, Secry. in Milk Co-op; one brother a full-time travelling agent
3	1	33	Murao	Owns a flour mill and an oil press
4	1	24	Murao	Owns a flour mill
5	1	21	Kalwar	Owns a sweets shop
6	1	12+1½+3/10	Murao and two Muslims	Combined ownership of flour and rice mills. The two Muslims are traders
7	1	16+11	Dhobi	One brother drives taxi in Delhi
8	1	21½	Dhobi	Permanent work (washerman's) and shop in Bombay
9	1	10	Chamar	Works in Kanpur in a leather factory

TABLE 10.4

Input and output: one Kb. plot of wheat*

Inputs		Cost (Rs.)
Seeds	- 10 kilos	20.00
Irrigation	- five hours by tubewell rented at Rs. 6 per hour	30.00
Labour (man-days)		
	Weeding - 8	
	ploughing - 4	
	harvesting - 4	
	threshing - 5	
	Wages at Rs. 2 per diem	42.00
Fertiliser (kilos):		
	DAP - 8	
	Potash - 6	
	Urea -13	28.60
	Total cost	Rs.120.60

Output** = 4 quintals (4 x 100 seers)		Earnings (Rs.)
a) Gross earnings at minimum government price[+] (Rs.105 per quintal)		420.00
	Net profit	299.40
b) Gross earnings at maximum government price[++] (Rs.175 per quintal		700.00
	Net profit	579.40

c) Wage as percentage of gross earnings at minimum price

$$= \frac{42}{420} \times 100 = 10\%$$

* The above data was provided by the family of the ex-*Taluqdar*, to whom I am grateful for allowing me access to their diary, which records the precise amounts of inputs as well as a daily record of work done on their land. The data relates to a 1 kb. plot left fallow from May - October. A new variety of wheat (RR-21) was grown from November to the following April. In this particular case it was found to be more remunerative to cultivate only one crop per year.

** Even in 1975 a plot with no regular irrigation or modern inputs yields less than 1 quintal per kb.

[+] Official government price.

[++] Price operating on open market.

the households own 20kb or more land and 74% of the households own 10kb or less (including 11% landless). The top 7% own 34.6% of the village land, whereas the bottom 63% (excluding 11% landless) own 43.5%.

In 1969, the first tubewell was installed by the ex-*taluqdar* family. By 1975, the number of tubewells had slowly risen to ten. The owners, apart from irrigating their own land, rent out their tubewells to the owners of neighbouring fields. Also, the number of improved, efficient Persian wheels had increased to six by 1975. This facilitates controlled, timely irrigation. Suddenly, productivity has increased several fold. The improvement in irrigation technology was soon followed by the introduction of new high-yielding variety seeds and chemical fertilisers, which further increased yields. With all these new inputs, if land is cultivated by hired labour the wages represent only 10% of the total output (at minimum price, for the major crop: wheat), whereas by leasing out land for sharecropping, the owner receives only 50% of the produce. Even after deducting the increased cost of the new inputs, the increase in productivity has been so great that the profits to the owner have increased immensely (see Table 10.4). A small family therefore no longer needs to lease out land because of lack of family labour.

Thus the changes in agricultural production have led to changes in the relations between different strata in the village. The ex-*taluqdar* family, who used to lease out all their land in the village (about 225kb) five years ago, now cultivates almost all of it by farm labour and casual wage labour. For example, from June 1, 1974 to April 11, 1975, 1,152 man-days of farm labour and 1,747 man-days of wage labour were thus employed. Within the village system, the ex-*taluqdar* family can be said to belong to the 'big landlord' stratum. The rest of the village households can be classified into four strata, according to landownership and landlessness. This is a simplified method of stratification but helps in understanding the changing interrelationships.

Rich Peasants	:	above 20kb of land
Middle Peasants	:	between 10 and 20kb
Small Peasants	:	less than 10kb
Landless	:	no land

I took a sample of 25 households (excluding the ex-*taluqdar* household and the landless households) to see the pattern of 'leasing in' or 'leasing out'[7] of land (see Table 10.5). The village as a whole has 63% small, 19.9% middle and 7% rich peasant households; 11% are landless. The sample has 56%, 36% and 8% respectively in these three strata. Out of 14 small peasant households, six do not rent or lease, three only rent

7. Hereafter referred to as 'renting' and 'leasing' respectively.

TABLE 10.5

Ramdaua sample households: renting and leasing of land

Sample households	Land (kbs.)			Pairs of bullocks owned
	owned	rented	leased	
1	1	8		1
2	1½			
3	2	7		½
4	2½		2	
5	2½		1½	
6	2½			
7	3½		3½	
8	3¾	½		2
9	4			1
10	5			
11	6¼		3¼	
12	6½			
13	7		7	½
14	7¾			
15	10½		4	
16	10¾		8¼	
17	11	15		1
18	11½	4		1
19	12¼			
20	14½			1
21	15		9½	
22	15½	1½		1
23	19	8		1
24	29¼		1¼	1
25	65		30	1

and five households lease land. Of nine middle peasant households, two do not rent or lease; four rent and three lease land; of the latter three households, one is comprised of only one adult male who works for the ex-*taluqdar* family, and another is comprised of two adult males, now growing old. The third household derives a significant amount of income from a washerman's job in Bombay and insufficient family labour is available for agriculture. Their reason given for leasing part of the land was its distance from their homes, and therefore their inability to supervise it. Finally, in the rich peasant stratum, both the households in my sample lease land. In one case, it is an insignificant proportion of the land owned and in the other case, the proportion of land leased has been declining over the last two years since the peasant acquired a tubewell.

Thus the pattern which emerges shows that the rich peasants are no longer inclined to lease land: instead they tend to cultivate their land with family and/or wage labour. The small peasants are beginning to lease land; lack of the basic means of production, like a pair of bullocks, is an important reason in this context. And middle peasants, who have the means of production and can afford to pay for irrigation and fertiliser, are renting land. Also, it can be anticipated that more and more small peasants will gradually lose their land due to poverty, debt, mortgage and, finally, foreclosure. The most frequent rate of interest for money is 50% per annum. For food loans the interest rate can be as high as 100%.

At this stage in the argument it is important to analyse the need for loans, which is the beginning of the process that could, ultimately, lead to the selling of land. If a seer (slightly less than a kilogram) of grain is accepted as a reasonable estimation of consumption per day for one consumption unit (see Table 10.6), then the annual grain requirement per consumption unit comes to 18.25km (one Kaccha Maund = 20 seers). In my sample only five (20%) out of the twenty-five households produce more than 18.25km per consumption unit (see Table 10.7). There are of course other sources of income, but this does at least give some indication of the extent of poverty and the need to borrow money or grain.

Here, I must mention another important economic category in the village. With the increase in productivity due to the introduction of tubewells and, consequently, new agricultural inputs, commerce has become very important. A few households, practising trade, fall into the stratum of rich peasants in terms of income, although they own very little or no land.

Another significant contribution to income comes from work outside the village. The majority of the people in this category migrate seasonally for a stretch of 15 days to a month, especially to the cities of Kanpur and Lucknow, where they do construction work or buy and sell old newspapers, empty cans and bottles etc. Others have permanent jobs, such as bus conductor, clerk, factory worker, washerman, Air Force technician and soldier. The majority of these migrants from village Ramdaua

TABLE 10.6

Index of consumption units*

Age group	Male/female	Consumption unit
0- 1	M/F	Zero
1- 5	M/F	0.30
5-10	M/F	0.50
10-20	F	0.70
10-20	M	0.75
20-45	F	0.85
20-45	M	1.00
45+	F	0.70
45+	M	0.80

* The index was compiled as a result of talking to a number of villagers about the relative food consumption by persons of different ages and sexes. Obviously, it does not apply accurately to each person in the village. It should be treated as a rough, average measure only.

TABLE 10.7

Grain production of sample households

Sample No.	Land Owned (kb.)	Total grain in a year * (km.)	Consumption Units	Grain produced per year per consumption unit (km.)	Buffaloes owned
1	1	38	4.55	8.351	
2	1½	4	4.55	0.879	
3	2	26	2.15	12.093	
4	2½	7.10	4.25	1.670	
5	2½	4.5	2.45	1.836	
6	2½	0.625	2.20	0.284	
7	3½	15.5	1.65	9.40	
8	3¾	45.75	4.85	9.432	
9	4	34	4.25	8.000	
10	5	11.5	1.50	7.666	
11	6¼	23.5	6.20	3.790	
12	6½	55.5	3.10	17.903	1
13	7	13.75	4.00	3.437	
14	7¾	42.75	2.60	16.442	
15	10½	47.5	4.00	11.875	1
16	10¾	22.5	1.00	22.5	
17	11	84.5	6.40	13.203	1
18	11½	41	6.5	6.307	2
19	12¼	76.25	5.30	14.386	
20	14½	46	5.40	8.518	
21	15	27.5	1.80	15.277	1
22	15½	132.5	4.95	26.767	1
23	19	87	3.85	22.597	
24	29¼	110	3.45	31.884	1
25	65	354.5	10.40	34.086	3

* 'Total grain in a year' is not the total grain produced in a year on owner's land. It represents the grain available in a year after taking into consideration the grain share on rented and leased land. One *kaccha maund* (Km.) is equal to 41.1 lbs or 18.7 kilos.

TABLE 10.8

Ramdaua migration 1974-75 by households*

Land-owned (Kb)	Permanent occupations	Seasonal
Landless	-	4
0 - 5	13	30
5 -10	9	5
10 -20	4	3
20 -50	3	-
50+	2	-

* These figures refer to the total village population. They do not include *permanent* in-migration or out-migration of households. Village households with male members in permanent jobs outside the village are included.

come from the small peasant stratum and most of them migrate seasonally (see Table 10.8). The richer strata, proportionately, tend to take up permanent jobs. This in turn is related to their higher educational levels.

The changes caused by the introduction of the new agricultural technologies imply, essentially, the alienation from land of more and more poor peasants. The number of households belonging to the small peasant and the landless strata is increasing. Due to the continuing decline in the availability of land for share-cropping, a large family inevitably entails fragmentation of land. Therefore these strata are forced to turn to the wage labour market, which already has a regional surplus. The development of the regional economy is extremely important for the village. If a region has developed services and an industrial sector to attract the surplus labour, then, apart from providing ready employment in those sectors, rural wages also increase. In such a case, a large family may not be undesirable. However, 90% of the population in district Hardoi is rural, and medium or large-scale industry is almost non-existent. Under such conditions, wages are extremely low. For example, in 1974-75 the daily wage rate for adult males was Rs.2, which could only buy a kilogram of wheat at peak prices. All these changes in productive relationships would seem to point to the disappearance of the rationale for having large numbers of children.

Fertility Behaviour

Changing Attitudes to Family Size

In 1975, many villagers - especially the younger ones - considered the ideal number of children to be three: two sons and a daughter. "At least two sons, because sons are like eyes. If one has two eyes, then one can continue to see even if one of them is damaged. But if this happens to a one-eyed man, he has only darkness in his life." Another man said that two or three children are enough: "Then they are like gold. Seven or eight are like pigs." A washerman, who works in Bombay and owns two acres of land, likened a family to agriculture. "If one has a small family then all the children can be brought up properly - well fed, well clothed, well educated. But children of a large family cannot be well looked after." He was implying that productivity in a small farm can be greater than that on large farms.

Generally, I found that people with large families, especially the poor, complained about the large number of children to be fed, clothed and married off. Therefore, when it comes to *attitude*, people do not want large families. But the actual planning of family size is another matter, as the following case illustrates.

Shiv Kumar has two acres of land; a total of four acres is cultivated by him together with his married brother and father.

CHART 10.1

Ramdaua 1974: Age/sex pyramid

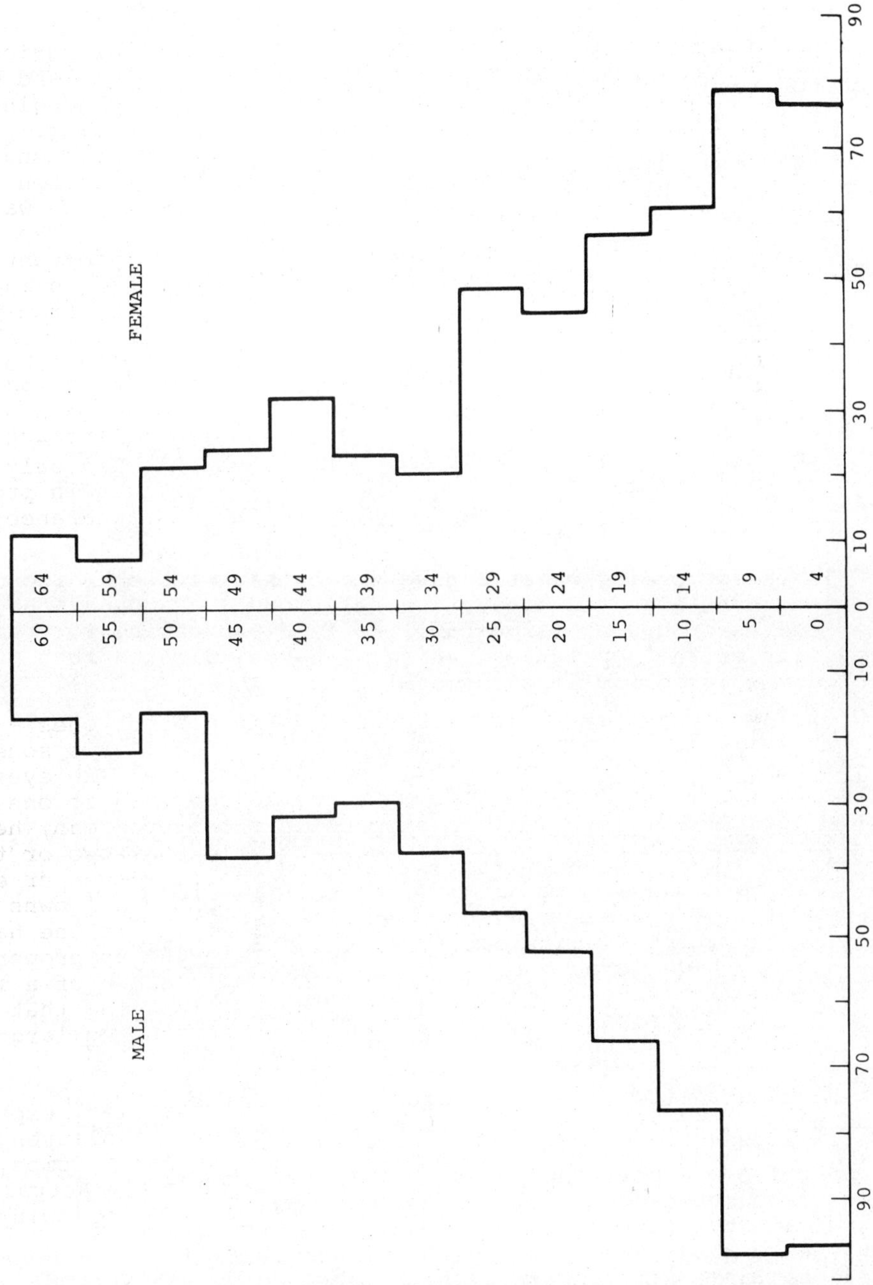

He is 29 years old and has four sons and a daughter. He used to pray to God, when he already had two sons and a daughter, not to give him any more children. "But God gave me more children - His wish." When I told him that now he had a large family and he was only 29 and asked him what he planned to do in the future, he replied: "Yes, I do not want any more children. I pray to God not to give me any more." Yet he did not want to be vasectomized.

Vasectomy is generally feared in village Ramdaua. A few years ago, a Family Planning 'camp' was organised in the region and two or three men, 'who could not escape', as the villagers put it, were forcibly taken in a police jeep and were vasectomized. During my visit in 1964-75 I personally met a young 25 year old bachelor who was one of the victims. Since then villagers equate family planning with forced vasectomy and tubectomy. There is no government plan filtering down to this village which involves *educating* and advising the villagers on family planning. Some men, especially the younger ones, know about condoms, but think using them is a tedious process. When I mentioned 'the pill' to them, they were quite excited about the idea. I wondered how the women would respond, but being a male myself, village women were not prepared to talk freely with me about contraception and I was therefore unable to discuss the pill with them.

In the preceding pages I have shown that with changing cultivation techniques and production relations in Ramdaua, the rationale for having large families is disappearing for the majority of the population. Also, I have indicated that people *do not want* large families anymore.

Finally, I have observed that despite the above two facts they are not, in practice, planning their family size. This apparent contradiction needs to be explained.

Constraint on Fertility Decline: Continued High Mortality

Village Ramdaua does not have a high net rate of population growth (1.15% per annum for the period 1961-73). While fertility is very high (Total Fertility Rate = 8.6) mortality is also relatively high (expectation of life at birth = 32 years; Infant Mortality Rate = 280 per thousand). This high fertility and mortality is reflected in the shape of the age pyramid (Chart 10.1), and the Child-Adult Ratio of 1.000.

High mortality rates generate a considerable element of risk and uncertainty about the survival of a child. It has already been noted that the new technologies and changing relations of production are bringing about the impoverishment of the landless labourers and the small peasants, which implies relatively more malnutrition and high mortality for the poor. Therefore they have good reason to try for higher fertility, which *may* lead to large family size. In the absence of any attempt by the government to counter the growing inequalities, it is hard to imagine a reduction in mortality. Consequently, a reduction in fertility cannot be expected for the majority of the population in village Ramdaua in the foreseeable future. Mortality decline is a necessary but not a sufficient condition for a decline in fertility. To look into the motivations for a potential decline in fertility, the labour market and the nature of employment opportunities should also be considered.

The above analysis shows that when large and increasing inequalities exist in agrarian structures into which new agricultural technologies have been introduced, and when additionally the regional economy is under-developed, a large family becomes undesirable. This is not to say that the development of services and an industrial sector necessarily leads to a desire for large families. But do we *want* to control only family size if by doing so the prevailing poverty and inequality remain unchanged?

We must realise that by defining the problem in terms of population *only* we are simply clouding the issue. The real problem emanates from the inequalities in the social structure and the extremely low standard of living of the majority of the population in an underdeveloped economy.

PART 4

PLANNING AND FERTILITY

CHAPTER 11

POPULATION PLANNING IN CHINA: THE INDIVIDUAL AND THE STATE

Three years after the founding of the People's Republic of China, the census showed a population of 582.6 million, with an annual growth rate of two per cent. The following year - 1954 - a research committee under the State Council was set up to look into the question of birth planning, and this was followed, two years later, by an Office of Birth Control, composed of representatives from the Ministries of Health, Propaganda, Culture and Commerce, as well as the Women's Federation, the Young Communist League and the Chinese Medical Association. Mao Tse Tung, while saying "we have this large population. It is a good thing" went on to add "this figure must also be of great concern to us all... The increase in grain harvest for the last two years has been 10,000,000 tons a year. This is barely sufficient to cover the needs of our growing population... Steps must therefore be taken to keep our population for a long time at a stable level, say, of 600,000,000".

Despite this statement, the programme had comparatively little effect, although it was followed by a Ministry of Health directive that "the government should take every step to guide the masses and meet their demands for birth control", as well as articles in such journals as Chinese Youth saying that birth control was good for the sake of both mothers and children. There were also exhaustive searches among traditional medicines for effective contraceptives - including the famous tadpole experiment. By 1958 the programme had lost all impetus: the Chinese deny that pronatalism ever became official policy but birth planning certainly ceased to be a major concern.

Lack of access to effective contraceptives was probably a secondary reason for the campaign's lack of success. The peasants were poor; children were a valuable source of future labour; women were still marrying young and few were educated. Land reform was not completed until 1952 and during the years of the first family planning campaign the vast mass of Chinese peasants was only gradually forming collectives and advanced collectives. The expansion of collectives into communes was largely a product of the Great Leap Forward.

The Great Leap Forward of 1968 both distracted attention from population questions and with its emphasis on small scale labour-intensive industry, especially rural industry, implied that a fast growing population could be absorbed. However, the Great Leap Forward itself proved to be over-ambitious and led, at least in the short term, to considerable confusion, which was intensified by the Russian withdrawal and the sequence of institutional changes and policy shifts which resulted.

In 1962 the second drive to contain population growth began. "Our emphasis on planned parenthood is entirely positive" said Chou en Lai. "Planned parenthood, where there is an increased production of goods and services, is conducive to raising people's standards of living". This second campaign encouraged contraception, sterilization for those who had completed their families, and toleration of abortion, as well as later marriage. The message ("Two children is just right, three is too many, four is a mistake") was carried to the people through every possible means: radio and newspapers, songs and entertainment, and the mobilization of cadres and intellectuals.

The mass line approach was apparently meeting with considerable success, and contraception was beginning to spread from the cities to the countryside, when the turmoil of the Cultural Revolution intervened. The questioning of established attitudes, combined with the lack of a single clear directive and the large numbers of unattached young people roaming the country, is thought to have led to a considerable rise in the birth rate. A graph of the birth rate in Tang Wen Commune, Shanghai county, provides some confirmation (see Chart 11.1).

But if the Cultural Revolution temporarily interrupted the emphasis on birth planning, it laid the foundation for much of the later successful campaign. There was renewed emphasis during the Cultural Revolution on the need for universal education - several elderly people the author met in China had learnt to read in the late Sixties - and the prospects for further education for the peasants improved as the result of criticism of the elitism of the universities. I asked an interpreter, Mr. Yao, who came from a peasant family, if his elder brothers had gone to university. He seemed surprised by the question. "Oh, no" he said "Before the Cultural Revolution it was almost impossible for people like us. I was lucky, because of my age, so that after the Cultural Revolution I was accepted".

As a direct result, medical care in the countryside improved. Medical education was shortened, and a large corps of barefoot doctors, working as peasants for part of their time, was created. The barefoot doctors helped not only to improve overall health in the communes, but to spread knowledge of contraception: of the seven chapters in their handbook, one is devoted to family planning and covers motivation and the importance of late marriage, as well as contraceptive methods.

To become a doctor today takes three years, the first year is a general course and the last two are divided between medical work in rural areas, and specialist subjects. Nurses undergo a two-year course and may become doctors after an additional six months training, while medical workers (such as barefoot doctors) have only a few months' basic training.

In the village there are health stations which give first aid, advice on preventive medicine and nutrition, and midwifery. In the cities, there are health centres run by residents' committees and staffed by older women who have retired from full-time work.

Of the small hospitals, the Pangpu neighbourhood hospital in a postwar overspill district of Shanghai was typical of several I saw. It carries out child welfare, acupuncture, obstetrics and gynaecology, X-rays and ENT. There are 24 doctors (six trained in traditional medicine) and 28 nurses and medical technicians. Of the total 52 medical personnel, two work in the country and 21 work outside the hospital in factories, schools and neighbourhoods. Bigger hospitals, like the Canton teaching hospitals, send medical teams to the countryside on a rotation basis to train barefoot doctors, advance the family planning programme (by carrying out sterilizations, for example), strengthen the rural health services and carry out propaganda for the 'patriotic public health campaign'.

Public health - preventive medicine and environmental hygiene - has been the major priority in China. Health education is partly directed to mobilizing the community for the effective disposal of refuse, latrine construction (nightsoil is still an important fertiliser but while it is stored and treated to destroy disease-carrying bacteria, the methane given off is now being tapped for fuel) and control of communicable diseases. Women are screened each year for cervical and breast cancer and special stress is placed on the protection of eyesight. (Eye exercises are carried out regularly at school and workers in factories doing fine work have a six instead of an eight hour day). It was noticeable at the schools I visited that every minor cut and graze was painted liberally with gentian violet.

Mothers are encouraged to breast feed, and home visits by medical workers teach desirable nutritional practice, and nutrition is also taught in school. Special efforts to involve grandmothers in nutrition education have been made, because of the influence that their beliefs and habits have on younger members of the family, and because it is thought that they have a store of useful experience.

An even more important aspect of the Cultural Revolution, perhaps, was the resulting change in people's attitudes. From it arose the campaign to criticise Confucius and Lin Piao, and the questioning of Confucianism has proved of particular relevance to the position of women.

Mrs. Chun is a good example of the increasing control women are able to have over their lives. She is the chairman of the revolutionary committee of an electronic appliance factory in Changsha, Hunan province. The child of poor parents, she became a street beggar at the age of seven. After the revolution, she married and became a housewife, and worked for a residents' organisation. "Then I thought, housewives must organise". In 1965, with three other women, she began to make paper string in half a room which had previously been a pigsty. A year later they switched to making radio transformers, and then condensers and 40 watt amplifiers.

CHART 11.1

Birthrate 1963-1974

Chart copied by author from wall of
Health Centre at Tang Wen People's Commune
Shanghai County (5400 households)

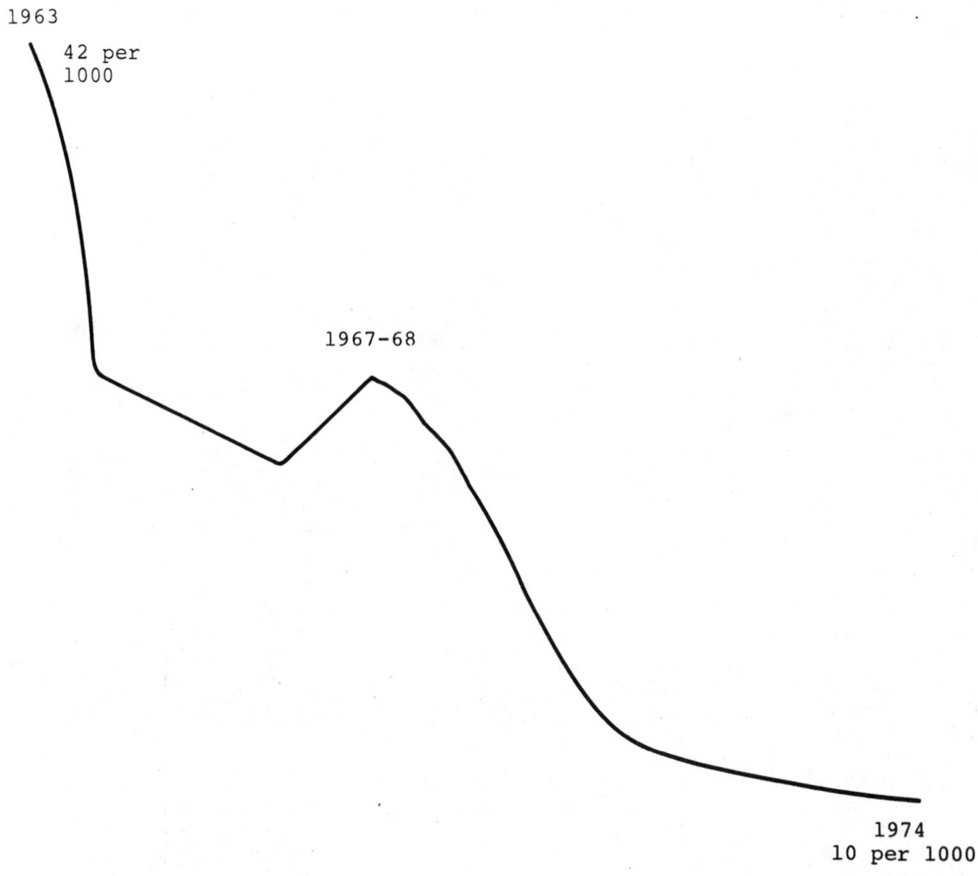

Today, there are 192 workers in the factory. The workers collected and saved sufficient funds for the new five-floor factory, deceptively hidden down a back street, and built it themselves, bricks and all. It is a housewives' factory, but provides employment for a substantial number of men as well - 'educated youth' and the mentally or physically disabled, who are unable to cope with the greater demands of, for example, a heavy industrial job. Last year the factory made 200,000 yuan for the State and kept over 100,000 in profit to plough back into expansion. "From controlling a small family" said Mrs. Chun, beaming, "I have come to organise a large one. In the old society, I could never dream of becoming a leader of a factory ..."

Mrs. Chun's story is not untypical. There are many women in more senior posts - a quarter of the delegates to the fourth Congress were women - and in more unusual roles. The vice-chairman of the revolutionary committee at the huge Nanking petrochemical plant we visited was a woman. But changes in the status of women are probably measured less by the activities of the comparatively few, however noticeable, in top positions, than by those of the mass of housewives and mothers.

Most women in China now seem to work, and much has been done to make this easier for them. Mrs. Wu, at Pangu neighbourhood explained:

> "Women of my age are generally employed. They no longer stay at home. Of the women living here, 70 per cent are cadres, and workers, in state-owned offices and enterprises. The remainder are organised into neighbourhood workshops. Formerly, people said a woman's place was in the home, looking after the kitchen and the children. Now, females in the home during the day are usually either old people or small children."

Those women whose family responsibilities make it impossible for them to work in an ordinary job now work in support services to enable other women to go to the factory or the field. They run neighbourhood shoe-mending services, laundries, and places for mending clothes, as well as take-away restaurants, creches and kindergartens.

Posters everywhere proclaim that women hold up half the sky, and that women can do anything men can do. The vast majority of children's stories show small female red soldiers doing anything from keeping the streets clean to outwitting and outfighting enemies of the people. The theme is repeated in films, puppet shows and operas: girls are the central characters and come triumphantly through every possible predicament.

As the representatives of the Women's Federation pointed out, real equality will take a long time to achieve. The Federation itself - like all the propaganda - is evidence that women still need special attention. It is a mass organisation with five specific tasks: to organise women for political study and to take an active part in movements such as that to criticise Confucius; to educate women to play a full role in production and all the other activities of the country; to discover and train women cadres; to look after the well-being and interests of women, and, finally, to educate women in internationalism.

Carrying out the fourth task- ensuring the well-being of women - involves seeing that women are specially cared for during the four periods (menstruation, pregnancy, childbirth and post-natal) when they are considered vulnerable, as well as helping to free them from housework so that they can do other things, and popularising family planning.

Some leading members of organisations, the Federation said, still prefer to give light jobs to women, with the concommitant low pay. Certainly there still seems to be confusion, in allotting work and work points, between large machines (even if easily operated) and heavy work. In the country, 56 days paid maternity leave is not yet universal, and work points are calculated on a system which means that women, being less strong, get less. Even in the model commune Tachai women do not get equal work points, because, it is said, much of the work still involves heavy labour like breaking granite. The mechanisation of agriculture should accelerate change here: a woman, they agree, can drive a tractor as well as a man. Women qualify for a retirement pension five years earlier than men.

The Cultural Revolution also led to a further shift towards the concept of developing an agrarian proletariat (heretical as it is to traditional Marxists, and as the Russians had in fact found it) and China's resources were ploughed into agricultural development rather than the creation of an industrial society. The general principle is of "taking agriculture as the foundation and industry as the leading factor" in developing the nation's economy.

This combination of industry and agriculture is a major theme in Chinese life. Efforts to raise the status of peasants, and to link agricultural workers to those in industry, start in the kindergartens. In Red kindergarten, Canton, not only are the three - to six-year old children taken to factories and communes to see how workers and peasants live, and learn from them, but they are actually taught to take part in agricultural labour and factory work themselves. There is a vegetable garden, which produces a considerable part of the school's food, and which the children cultivate. One class period a week is spent on work for which they have a contract with a local factory.

Older children, like those at the Hungwei Primary School in Kewilin, in the autonomous region of Kwangsi, besides making matchboxes and packing detergent powder into boxes under contract to local factories, have connections with two production brigades. Hungwei Primary School is in the middle of the town, so that most of the children do not come from an agricultural background, but are the sons and daughters of workers.

Divisions are further broken down by the use of part-time teachers in the school; workers and peasants who, in addition to their ordinary tasks, do some regular extra service. At Hungwei, these barefoot teachers were a quarter of the total staff.

Education to the age of 15 is now universal in China, but in the cities it is 17. The country areas are trying to raise the school leaving age, and in the various communes I visited, between 40 and 60 per cent now stay on for the extra two years, although this puts great demands on limited resources.

Those urban children who have an extra two years' schooling are described as 'educated youth'. When they leave school, they are assigned to work, and inevitably most of them are placed in communes. University education is only possible after 2-3 years' work and the numbers sent to the country are enormous. At the Double Bridge commune, outside Peking, the 40,000 inhabitants included 3,000 educated youth. Middle school graduates at the Tao Loi commune in Kwantung province had literally changed the face of the land in the last year, building 2,000 terraces and planting them with young fruit trees.

In addition to physical labour they bring the benefits of their greater education, for school courses combine the practical with theory. The educated youth can thus contribute scientific agricultural methods to the commune, and add, for example, to the resources of the agricultural research station which every commune seems to have. About a month each term they and their teachers go out to 'their' production brigades, transplanting rice, sowing seed and spreading manure. Every child becomes - at least in part - a peasant: every child is - in part - a worker.

Their labour is not viewed primarily as an addition to the country's productivity. At a truck factory in Nanking I was told by Mr. Lin, the director of the office of the factory's revolutionary committee, that they generally have a hundred or more middle school children working there at any one time. When asked how efficient they were, he said "We do not regard them as a labour force. We are training them to understand the workers and to become the successors in producing a socialist country."

The Chinese have achieved a social security framework of schooling, health, security in old age and employment which has transformed the life of the agricultural worker. Mr. Li, at the Tao Loi commune, said that while the standard of living is not high, everybody has sufficient for a plain life - which includes such 'luxuries' as bicycles, watches, radios and sewing machines - and the 67,000 commune members had savings of 1.6 million yuan (for an indication of what this means, the average industrial income is around 60 yuan a month).

The demarcation between urban and rural communities is in any case decreasing: the communes are no longer purely agricultural. The Double Bridge Commune has 15 enterprises including flourmills and machinery workshops; 30 per cent of the commune's income comes from industry. The Tao Loi commune has eight factories producing lime, cement, machinery, plastic tools; the Tangwen commune, which receives 35 per cent of its income from its nine factories, produces among other things agricultural machinery, tools and furniture.

The structure of the communes means that they are able to finance quite large local projects, such as electrification, as well as to provide the labour to carry out the necessary terracing, canal and dam work. Collective labour has lessened the need for any individual family to have several sons, as well as providing a means of carrying out developments like grain storage and afforestation, which protect the peasant from unpredictable nature. "We are the masters now; we decide the way things will go" is a common phrase in China today, and is apparently a totally satisfactory answer to questions as diverse as how the factory worker will cope with mechanisation without succumbing to the alienation of the conveyor belt, and how an elderly hotel cook sums up the effect of the revolution on himself.

Mrs. Tang, of the Double Bridge Commune outside Peking, was the member responsible for family planning in the women's organisation there. She said there were five such people in charge of five sections of her little village. Each had just over ten women to supervise. "We tell them the situation as it is today. Now that political consciousness has been raised, people understand that two children are enough - even if neither is a boy". Mrs. Tang has three children "I didn't teach myself well enough") but said that now in her village every eligible woman was using family planning - mainly IUDs or pills. She tells young couples of the benefits of deferred marriage and said that there was a close connection between deferred marriage and successful family planning.

Mrs. Tang's home, though barer than the town dwellings, contained a radio and a sewing machine. It was four roomed, with a traditional kang which uses hay, straw and coal for fuel, and she was clearly proud of it. In the past, she said, the local houses had been one or two roomed and made of mud. She and her husband saved for two years to buy the bricks and other building materials, while they lived with their parents, and then the village built the house in one day.

At the Changsha housewives' factory, the person responsible for family planning was also the Chairman of her branch of the Woman's Federation. She said that for better birth control it was necessary to explain that with two children women have more time and energy to work for the state and that they can liberate themselves and their families.

In her neighbourhood, men marry around the age of 26, women around 24. Once a couple have their first child they wait four to six years before having a second. They use pills, IUDs, abortion and sterilisation - both male and female, although the proportions are around 70:30 respectively.

In Kweilin, in the Kwangsi autonomous region, down on the Vietnam border, women seem to delay marriage still further - from 26 to 28 - and again aim for a two child family. Kwangsi is unusual among the autonomous regions because it is not sparsely populated and it has therefore been fully involved in the birth planning campaigns, which, I was told, have been effective in the country districts as well as in Kweilin itself. One young woman to whom I spoke said she had several boyfriends who regarded her as a possible partner before she married a local boy with whom she had fallen in love. She was then 23 and they waited almost another three years to marry. She had two small children (which were not breastfed, her mother took over feeding and caring for the babies as soon as she came out of hospital) and she said that once she had her first, she had wanted no more children - she had not realised what problems they caused. But she used no contraception after the birth of the first child. Now, her husband uses contraception. He also did the shopping and much of the cooking which was usually carried out on a Sunday; during the rest of the week they ate at work or his mother bought food from the takeaway shops.

In the older parts of the towns, houses are arranged around a courtyard. I visited a home in Peking belonging to an elderly couple, whose married son and daughter-in-law also lived there. The lady, who was 60, worked in a production group making clothes, while her husband worked on a forest farm and came home once a week. He had been a rickshaw puller in the old days and sometimes he earned enough money for them to eat; sometimes not. She was then a servant. In recent years she has learned to read.

The little house was comfortable and seemed to have most of the basic amenities, though water was provided by a tap in the courtyard. Three of the family are working in State industry and so get heating allowances in the winter in addition to their pay; they eat around one kilo of meat a week and save 40-50 yuan a month. The son is a welder and the daughter-in-law works in a carpet factory; they were 27 and 26 when they married.

Courtyards such as these, which usually contain some 5 to 15 households, offer an additional level of medical care, in the person of a courtyard orderly, who, besides learning basic first aid and nutrition, is also responsible for spreading awareness of the benefits of birth planning and for helping to reinforce the regularity with which contraceptives are used.

Much of the credit for what is generally admitted to be an extremely successful campaign to control population growth must go to the administration and the comprehensive nature of the programme itself. At every level of every organisation there is a member responsible for family planning: the woman in the factory is propagandised not only by one of her fellows in the work unit (around 15 people) under the overall guidance of the union

TABLE 11.1

Fertility figures, Pangpu neighbourhood
January - September 1975

Total fertile women	3376
sterilized	1438
pill	735
injections	69
IUD	200
diaphragm	319
lactating	22
waiting for baby	379
widowed	27
divorced/separated	6
infertile	63
menopausal	85

or the Women's Federation, but by her street committee or courtyard orderly. Her husband will face similar pressures at work and in the neighbourhood, and both of them will meet yet other responsible persons in their discussion groups and in the course of any other activities they undertake. It is apparent that the Chinese are unconcerned about any overlap of effort when you realise that the average couple may encounter persuasion from five or six different sources, each of which is responsible for no more than around 20 people.

Administratively this does not seem to lead to lack of efficiency. In Tangwen People's commune, the returns from each brigade to July 1975 had been entered on an elaborate wallchart in the hospital. Dr. Han's hospital had the fertility figures for the 13 residents' groups in the area covered by her hospital, totalled to September 1975, when I visited her in November.[1] The visit had not been scheduled, so that the figures could not have been specially prepared (see Table 11.1). When I complimented Dr. Han, and asked how she managed to achieve such excellent reporting, she said only that "we have to rely on the people ... China, it seems, has gone far in convincing the people that individual decisions and choices have a public impact". As the Women's Federation put it: "The interests of the State are closely linked with those of private families. The State has to make a general plan, while each area and each family makes its own plan".

The people have learned to plan for themselves and to plan for the future, and now see the planning of births as a perfectly logical part of this process. Family planning strategy is subordinate to overall planning, and arises naturally out of complete plans for the economy, for agriculture, and for development. The greater level of political consciousness among the mass of the Chinese since the Cultural Revolution means that this planning is understood right down to the individual level.

Individuals see their fertility plans as an integral part of the plan for their area, affecting not only birth rates but how the community's funds can be deployed and what priorities will have to be for the future. All of them, at the annual accounting period, are involved in such planning, and the decentralised nature of the funding for even quite major projects means that the demographic imperatives in choosing priorities are easily recognised.

---

1. My visit to China, for three weeks in November, 1975, was partly sponsored by the Helen Seymour Memorial Fund and the Simon Population Trust.

CHAPTER 12

FROM 'ACCOMMODATION' TO 'INTERVENTION':[1] SOCIO-ECONOMIC HETEROGENEITY AND DEMOGRAPHIC PATTERNS

> "Unless the peculiarities and differences of the ways by which various sub-populations of a nation are affected by population change are well understood and explicated, action to deal with population problems will fail to acquire the natural constituencies on whose support it should vitally depend."[2]

INTRODUCTION

The papers presented in this volume are the results of studies which have been conducted with precisely the objective in mind which Demeny singles out as one of the most important aspects of population policies, namely to disaggregate the available macro-demographic data and try to understand the rationale behind the fertility behaviour displayed by different sections of the population.

In this chapter I attempt not only a cross-cultural synthesis of the data and hypotheses suggested by each of the eight micro-studies, but also to provide a theoretical framework for handling such diverse data.

There are a few precedents of this type of cross-cultural analysis, but most of them lack the necessary integrated research base. Molnos, for instance, examined a series of studies geared to throw light on fertility behaviour and concluded 'that they were non-comparable and repetitive' (1971:64).

---

1. The relationship between individuals and their physical environment is an age old concern: "The three point range of variation in the man-nature orientation: Subjugation to Nature, Harmony with Nature, and Mastery over Nature is too well known from the works of philosophers and culture historians to need much explanation" (Kluckholn and Strodtbeck, 1973:13). In this paper the concept is broadened to include social relationships, and as such is applied to help explain fertility behaviour.
2. Demeny, 1974:61.

By contrast I regard our eight studies not only as truly comparable but also as complementary.[3] Their overall analysis presents an intellectual challenge which I here attempt to meet.

Until not so long ago population growth in Third World countries attracted attention solely for its apparently unfavourable impact on capital formation in particular, and economic growth in general (e.g. Coale and Hoover, 1958). It is only recently that the mutual interdependence between a group's fertility and its total environmental situation has come to be fully appreciated. This realisation has opened up a whole new area of investigation: rather than treating Third World fertility behaviour as a factor which can be explained in isolation from the socio-economic context in which it takes place, population growth rates are now regarded as a reflection of other phenomena.

The 'demographic transition' in developed countries denotes the transition from 'high to low levels of both birth and death rates, with an intervening period of relatively rapid population growth while death rates declined before birth rates followed... The factors commonly adduced in explanation of the changes in vital rates are mainly of the kind which accompany industrial development and rising standards of living' (Cassen, 1972:2). The corresponding changes which occurred during the last century in developed countries between the process of industrialisation and 'modernisation' on the one hand, and demographic changes on the other, are often taken to provide population growth models for present day Third World countries. However, a mere statistical correlation does not necessarily represent a causal relationship, nor can it explain the reason for such a relationship, even if it does exist.

Now that Third World population growth has come to be treated as a dependent variable, attempts are being made to establish the nature of the determining variables. Since there are a large number of different variables that affect population growth, most of which are extremely difficult to quantify, many economists and socio-demographers are tempted to abstract from the complex reality and build models by attributing growth rates to the operation of one, or a few, specific variables - assuming a *ceteris paribus* clause. Thus while one argues on the basis 'that parents assume an expected level of support from any child born'

---

3. This is probably the result of our project design which had built into it from its inception a comparative and complementary approach, unlike many other cross-cultural research projects which try to synthesize *post facto* the diverse findings produced by different field-work and which lack a common denominator. Such attempts have often proved frustrating and futile. The advantages of carefully pre-planned cross-cultural research are further exemplified in the interesting findings of Arnold, et al., 1975.

(Chernichovsky, 1975:8), others suggest cost/benefit analyses of children (Becker, 1960). 'There is one school of thought that emphasises the inverse relationships found between levels of education (and possibly of nutrition and health) and family size ... Another school of thought emphasises incentives and disincentives' (Edwards, 1974:19).

All these different analyses - and many more could be cited - try to treat only one of the many aspects of fertility behaviour in isolation from the total complex of relevant variables. This is a far too simplistic approach to one of the most vital factors of human existence. For society as a whole, it is essential to reproduce itself, a fact which seems to be frequently overlooked in discussions relating to fertility behaviour. Bearing in mind the central importance of fertility for all living things, the papers presented here suggest that a 'demographic transition' in the Third World can result only when the majority of people are in a position to exert a determining influence not only over their own socio-physical environment, but also over the lives of their children - when they have options and can make choices meaningful to them. This, it would appear, cannot be expected to occur by manipulating one, or even a few socio-economic variables in an attempt to affect fertility behaviour. A radical re-structuring of social systems seems to be a necessary precondition of successful fertility control. This argument rests on our findings, which though provisional, clearly indicate that only those individuals and sections of society who are in a position to influence their own lives can be expected to develop an *interventive* approach. They are likely to become concerned with the kind of life they can secure for their offspring and consequently consider planning the size of their families.

Our eight micro studies, which range across Asia and Africa, indicate that until very recently large numbers of children were of vital importance in the people's struggle for survival. For instance, in Ramdaua, a village in Uttar Pradesh, India, it is no more than six years ago that conditions began to change in this respect. A number of interdependent reasons explain the need for high fertility, while rural communities were largely 'closed systems'.[4] Though I discuss these variables below I want to stress here that I am not doing so in order to examine the possible relationship between changes in one or more of them on the one hand and corresponding changes in fertility behaviour on the other, which is frequently the object of such an

---

4. Though the myth of the existence of completely isolated and self-sufficient small societies has long been exploded, it is still meaningful to distinguish between 'closed communities' which have only marginal contact with the outside world and are group-introverted (Srinivas, 1955), and 'open communities' which are fully integrated in the wider society and have a broader horizon.

CHART.1

Traditional Ecology - high fertility

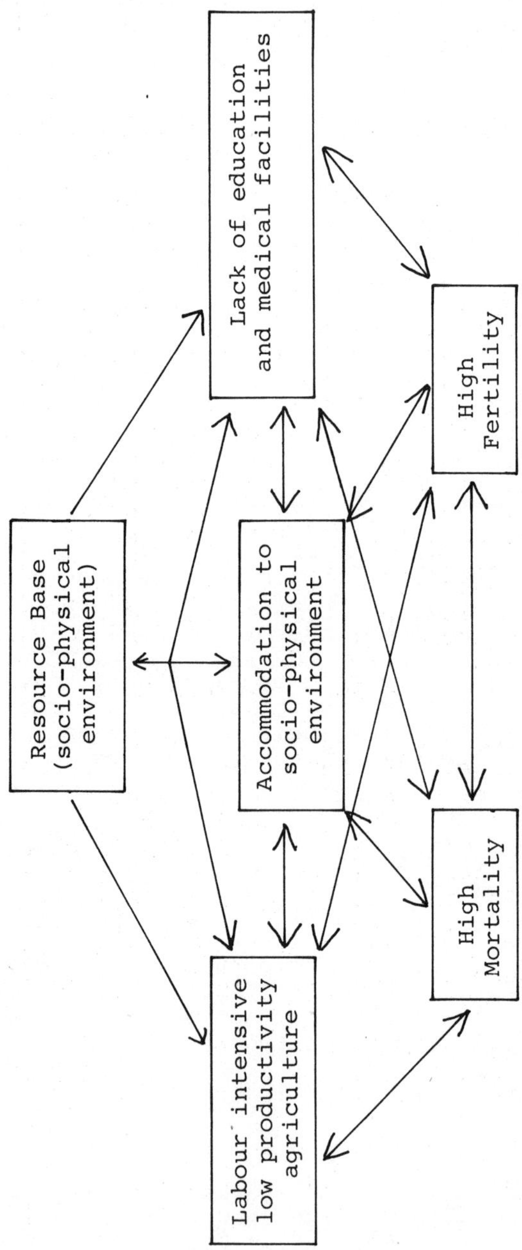

exercise. By way of contrast I try to use this examination as a means of showing the intricate complex of variables which affects the relationship between groups of people and their socio-physical environment (see Chart 12.1) and which is reflected in their fertility behaviour.

Closed Rural Communities - Accommodation to Socio-physical Environment[5]

Most of these communities had little contact with the outside world and little control over their environment; they were largely subject to the hazards of nature which perpetually threatened the individual family's livelihood and the whole group's survival. Under these conditions, several factors operate which necessitate high fertility. High levels of mortality, particularly infant mortality, which still pertain among large sections of the Third World, put a premium on high fertility. Since one of the central objectives of life is to ensure the continuation of the species, societies which fail to meet this need obviously decline and ultimately die out. This fundamental human response to threats of extermination by famine and sickness is exemplified in the fact that the one society among the eight we studied which shows the highest mortality also has the highest fertility (see Chapter 10). This does not necessarily imply that a reduction in mortality will by itself result in declining fertility, which is evidenced by the example of the Wataita in Kenya who have a lower mortality but the highest standardised mean number of living children per woman among the eight societies we studied (see Chapter 9).

Their limited technological know-how put these closed rural communities largely at the mercy of nature and was responsible for a high degree of risk in their lives. With irregular rainfall, recurrent droughts or floods and high levels of mortality, it is extremely difficult for a family or group of families to ensure a reasonable level of living for the present, let alone plan for the future. Traditional agriculture, moreover, is highly labour intensive. Therefore, large families were an advantage, particularly in areas with a low man/land ratio where additional household labour facilitated the expansion of the area under cultivation.

The detailed account of the labour intensity of traditional agricultural production in Ramdaua shows how large numbers of

---

5. 'For example, an authentic TBA (Traditional Birth Attendent) may take it for granted that a relatively large family is a mark of divine favour, or that it is imprudent to do anything (such as use an IUD) that could deprive the body of its state of harmony with nature. Ideas like these do not seem absurd in societies where accommodation to the environment in traditional ways may still seem the feasible strategy' (Simons, 1975).

children enabled families to get larger areas under share-cropping tenancies. Landlords shrewdly realised that tenants with more household labour provide a larger yield than those with small families (see p. 191).

On the basis of our studies in Kenya we can help to explain the need for large numbers of sons as a means of the family's protection amidst a state of continuous warring. The traditional settling pattern among the Maragoli, where a man arranged for the households of his sons to surround and protect the parent unit, is an adaptive response to a hostile social environment and also inevitably encourages high fertility. The lack of literacy and the inability to produce lasting assets among many African tribal societies may be a contributory factor in their attempt to achieve parental immortality by means of having many offspring.

These conditions of extreme uncertainty, which were part of the life of the majority of families living in 'closed rural communities', make realistic planning for the future impossible for tenants in particular and clients in general. This is not to say that these people led a hand-to-mouth existence unconcerned about the future. All I am trying to stress here is the low level of technological know-how and poverty for the many, which restrained them from protecting themselves against major environmental hazards such as droughts and floods, and doomed them to life-long client status. Their large numbers of children were not the result of anything even remotely approaching cost/benefit considerations but were rather the result of a necessary part of the process of adaption to environmental conditions. Families were not concerned with the cost of additional children but regarded them as an essential part of their lives, and as a means to satisfy many of their unconscious and subconscious needs. They had no option but to accommodate to their socio-physical environment. This is often reflected in traditional beliefs such as the ancestor worship in Africa (see p. 71) and the Karma concept in Sri Lanka (see p. 147).[6]

From Closed to Open Community - From 'Accommodation' to 'Intervention'

As already mentioned the exposure of previously closed communities to exogenous 'modernising' influences is only a very recent phenomenon in all the eight societies we studied.

---

6. In Spanish American attitudes toward illness and death one finds the same submission to superior powers. 'If it is the Lord's will that I die, I shall die' is the way they express it, and many a Spanish-American has been known to refuse the services of a doctor because of this attitude (Kluckhohn, 1973:13).

Medical facilities, which were among the first technological innovations, helped to reduce the incidence of epidemics, such as smallpox and plague which used to be rampant and had caused many deaths; malaria, another major threat to human life, has almost been eradicated. Even villages remote from health centres, such as for instance Umueke in the East Central State of Nigeria, experience at least some of the benefits from modern medicines (see p. 79). The resulting decline in mortality and raising of the expectancy of life, without a concomitant decline in fertility, is the basic cause of the population problem. The rapidly growing numbers soon result in population pressing on limited landed resources. For instance, the Maragoli now occupy the most densely populated area in Kenya and have the highest man/land ratio among the eight societies we studied. 'A topic of major concern in developing country demography today is the relation between birth and death rates. It is argued that parents are interested not so much in having babies as in having surviving children, and, therefore, that decline in mortality is a necessary, although not a sufficient condition for declining fertility. The insufficiency of the condition may be seen from the fact that many countries have had 50 years or more of significant mortality decline, with little change in fertility' (Cassen, 1973:3). Though many countries have failed to show significant fertility declines in line with falling mortality rates, this does not necessarily mean that there have been no such changes among some of the sub-populations involved. Macro-demographic data needs to be disaggregated before one can hope to begin to understand the differential fertility motivations for the various sub-strata of a country's population.

The opening up of 'closed communities' induced and/or furthered the process of internal socio-economic differentiation. Formal education seemed to provide the stepping stone for getting onto the first rung of the ladder to success. Among the Maragoli, for instance, the first generation of innovators - a small proportion of the community - took advantage of some of the modern educational facilities, and the new agricultural technologies. In doing so they discontinued many of their traditional extended family ties and moved to the roadside, where they built permanent houses, in contrast to the customary thatched roofed mudhuts. This 'roadside ecology elite' managed to raise their standard of living considerably: they have electricity, telephones, piped water etc. They began to feel that they were masters of their own fate and what is even more important they started planning the future of their children. They spent a lot of money to get their children through higher education (see p. 63). Our studies illustrate that education is a luxury which only the wealthier can afford. In India 'according to the 1971 census, of the population above 15 years 67 percent are illiterate, eight percent are literate without formal education, and only seven percent are matriculates or have higher qualifications' (Bardhan, 1974:70). In Kenya, where the law stipulates that primary education is free, it still requires a considerable cash expense to put children through their first years of schooling, quite apart from the opportunity cost involved (see Table 3.8).

The 'Maragoli Roadside Elite' radically changed their traditional ecology: from feeling powerless *vis-a-vis* the hazards of nature they began to be able to plan not only their own lives but even those of their children. These new horizons, however, did not immediately affect their fertility behaviour; they had almost as many children as their traditional counterparts, though some of them practised terminal birth control by means of sterilisation. By contrast, their children - the young professionals - display considerable change in their fertility, which has drastically declined: the marriage age of the daughters of the elite has been raised - the girls train as teachers, secretaries or nurses until they are in their late twenties and the young married couples, most of whom live in Nairobi, use contraception to have fewer and better-spaced children.

Thus a new 'cultural inventory' is a necessary precondition to planned fertility. It seems that only when people have alternative options among which to choose that they begin to be in a position to calculate their comparative chances of success. Only then are their hopes and aspirations raised and they start worrying about the quality of life their children are likely to have. Aspirations are an important variable in the process of modernisation and by changing group norms have a decisive impact on fertility behaviour (see p. 99).

The effect of changed aspirations on fertility is particularly noticeable in Sri Lanka. Though there is only little observed difference in the fertility behaviour between the different socio-economic strata, each of them appears to be differently motivated to limit the size of their families: the wealthiest are concerned with the way they can secure a bright future for their descendants. For the middle-strata the educated unemployment acts as a deterrent to have more children and even the poorest are sufficiently alert to be able to weigh up the odds of their children being able to make a living if they produce more than just two or three (see p. 169).

Sri Lanka's comparative success story against a background of economic difficulties is somewhat reminiscent of the incidence of the one-child system in parts of Hungary, which was first noticed during the early part of the 19th century. In this context 'evidence points to the paramount importance of economic aspirations - especially the desire to acquire, to hold on to and to accumulate land under the increasingly adverse combination of growing population pressures, stable or expanding latifundia and limited availability of alternative employment opportunities' (Demeny, 1972:171). Andorka, who carefully studied the literature relating to the Hungarian one-child system, confirms that the most reasonable explanation, which now seems to be generally accepted, lies in the then existing economic stagnation, which threatened a decline in the standard of living unless the total ancestral property could be passed on to a single heir. The cause of the one-child-system was thus a material one; not poverty but the fear of poverty (Andorka,

CHART 12.2

Modern ecology - planned fertility

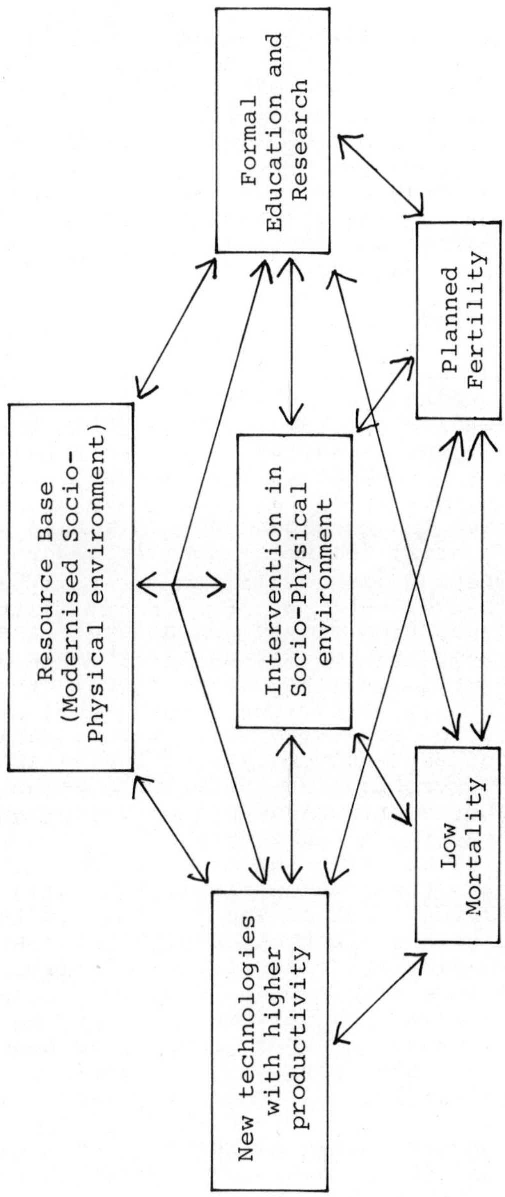

1969:13). These Hungarian peasants of the early 19th century practised family size control by induced abortion, infanticide, coitus interruptus and other means (Andorka, 1969:20). They developed a special moral code, which sanctioned the one-child system 'if a woman remained sterile, she was sympathised with; if she had no living children it was said it is her concern; but if a woman had more than two children, she is ridiculed, despised, condemned: 'can she not care?' or 'I would be ashamed if I littered as much' and the mother or mother-in-law generally knows the proper time to recommend it is better to wash the sheeting than the baby's napkin' (Andorka, 1969:21).

These Hungarian peasants obviously examined the chances of a good life for following generations if each couple produced more that one or two children and decided that it was best to keep their families small. 'We do not make beggars - said a young peasant ... The country is full of unemployed people ... They should give us land and land will produce people' (Andorka, 1969:14). Like their present-day Sri Lankan counterparts, these peasants practising the one-child system reduced their fertility because of their concern for the sort of life their children would be able to lead. They were in a position to influence their environment in such a way as to secure a reasonable standard of living for themselves and therefore also planned the numbers of children they produced. This displays an interventive approach, in contrast to the dependency on nature as well as on their patrons which still features among large proportions of Third World dwellers.

Kenya's rapid population growth can be explained by the fact that large sections of its population have so far hardly been affected by any modernising influences. For instance, the Wataita want many children (more sons than daughters!) because they need their help to cope with their labour intensive agricultural production. Yet only very few Wataita are able to produce sufficient crops to meet their own household's consumption needs; they therefore depend on cash earnings outside their subsistence farming to make up the deficiency. The upper strata among the Wataita, like the Maragoli Roadside Elite, use education to get onto the upward spiral; the higher the education and the higher the level of income of an individual, the greater appears to be her/his concern with the cost of educating children and the smaller the size of their families. Modernisation breaks the vicious circle of poverty for those who manage to get access to the new technologies, and sets up a new network of inter-relationships between demographic, economic, environmental and social variables effecting an overall, interventive approach (see Chart 12.2).

By contrast the poorer Wataita, in their endeavours to have at least one son who will make his way in life, produce many children to increase their own chance of success. With an inheritance system according to which each son gets an equal share of the ancestral estate, the small landholdings of the poorest become so fragmented over two or three generations that the individuals are forced to sell out and join the growing numbers of landless labourers (see p. 177). Among the Waitaita all illegitimate sons are automatically landless, and the number of illegitimate births is increasing. The raising of the age at which girls marry in Kenya does not result in their reduced fertility. Unlike in rural India and Sri Lanka where pre-marital sex relations are regarded as immoral and hardly any children are born outside wedlock, among some of the Kenyan tribes - certainly among the Wataita - a girl's virginity seems of little importance and no stigma is attached to pre-marital pregnancies, even though they may not be welcomed by the individual girls concerned. The infanticide of illegitimate babies indicates an as yet unmet, but felt, need for preventing the birth of potentially disadvantaged children.

The poorest among the Wataita and the Maragoli 'Traditional Ecological Stratum' suffer extreme deprivations. They face slow starvation regularly between February and May each year. Customary cultural practices and beliefs among them still regulate the interaction with their socio-physical environment; similarly they also affect their fertility behaviour. They have a high infant mortality as well as a high fertility rate. The solutions to problems of infertility are usually those provided by the traditional cultural inventory such as beliefs in sorcery or witchcraft. This traditional cultural store house of solutions, however, does not include any guidelines or provisions of how to deal with excessive fertility. This does not imply that traditional societies did not know how to avoid having undesirable additions to their numbers - they did practise abortion and infanticide - but usually only in cases of special social categories; e.g. when a couple broke the incest taboo. It simply means that until not so long ago the society as a whole was not really faced by the problem of excessive numbers. As already mentioned this is a fairly recent phenomenon. Those many among the Wataita and Maragoli who have gained little or no access to modern technologies and educational facilities, continue to operate with their customary 'cultural inventory'. They are so poor that they often do not know how to meet tomorrow's needs, let alone plan further ahead. They regard children as God's gift and continue to have as many as they can get. This is a logical consequence of their overall 'accommodation' to difficult environmental conditions. Their limited horizons prevent individual couples from realising that they will all be worse off if each of them produces large numbers of children. After all, the productivity of their labour is determined by the population/resource ratio of the larger economic environment, over which they themselves have no significant control; 'in other words, it depends on the general demographic and economic conditions obtaining outside the individual family, not on the size of that particular family. Certainly, the situation might improve if *every* family were to limit the number of its children, but in the absence of this it is possible that individual parents may derive relative economic benefit from producing large numbers of children in direct conflict with the needs of the economy as a whole' (White, forthcoming).[7]

The large number of rural Indian households who live below the poverty line are similarly caught in the paradox of family size. Here it is appropriate to recount an incident which I experienced when I visited Jairath in Ramdaua. I heard and watched the wailing of a young mother whose six month old baby had been taken by a wolf from her side while she was asleep during the previous night; in the morning all that could be found of the baby was half its head. I am relating this episode here not so much to arouse sympathy for these poor villagers but rather as a means to illustrate to people who are used to being able to exercise control over their environment that they belong to the privileged few. The majority of Third Worlders are still subject to the hazards of their socio-physical environment. In order to survive they must accommodate to their hostile surroundings.

The poor appear to be caught in a vicious circle of having difficulty of access to education and modern technologies, which puts them at the mercy of their social and physical environment and in turn is reflected in their 'accommodating approach', which prevents them from any attempt to plan the lives of their children and results in high fertility and so on. It is hardly reasonable to expect that this vicious circle can be broken at its 'fertility link' which is its most crucial one because it meets the ultimate objective of life. To expect this would in fact imply putting the onus of introducing a change on to the individual poor themselves, who in other contexts are recognised as needing most exogenous help (Chenery, 1974).

External intervention, in the form of modernising rural development and in particular bringing education and improved health to the mass of the people (Cassen, 1975:66), seems a much more strategic point at which to try and break into this vicious circle. Improvement in the levels of living of the poorest, who form a considerable proportion of the Third World population, is a necessary pre-condition of their entire participation in shaping their own as well as their children's lives. This in turn is a necessary pre-condition of fertility decline.

The apparent success in controlling the population growth in the People's Republic of China provides support for this proposition.[8] The revolution changed the socio-economic structure of Chinese society and enabled all sections to share not only the product of their labour but also the responsibilities of organisation and decision making. 'The people have learned to plan

---

7. This conflict is discussed in detail in Epstein & Jackson (eds.), The Paradox of Poverty (1975), Macmillan, India.
8. China's experience in population planning is so relevant to our 'Cross-cultural Study of Population Growth and Rural Poverty' that we were pleased when Penny Kane agreed to contribute a chapter on this topic to this volume.

for themselves and plan for the future, and now see the planning of births as a perfectly logical part of this process' (see p.207). To create public awareness of the problems resulting from unplanned population growth the State used a three part strategy; 'an extensive educational and propaganda campaign making use of village - and community-level party cadres to transmit and justify its policy objectives; and an effective free delivery system for family planning services, integrated into the health care system. The third component, apparently considered essential to the programme's success, is the active stimulating of intra-village antinatalist social pressures' (McNicoll, 1975:15). 'Birth planning education is always related to other factors in China and learned in the context of overall needs and policies' (Leonard, 1974:18). Every Chinese adult - man and woman - is a member of a study group, which meets regularly, sometimes as frequently as three times a week. These study groups enable individuals to keep informed about latest scientific advances which concern them and also to suggest areas where more research is needed; they also discuss fertility decisions.

In China's effort to disseminate information and encourage a positive response to population policies, the effective agent is personal contact. 'Nearly every child in China now has a course on conception and contraception and the reasons for birth planning and delayed marriage as part of a course in physiology given the last year of middle school (i.e. the 9th and last year of universal education)' (Leonard, 1974:15). The 'barefoot doctors' (herbalists) carried the main responsibility for birth education, among Chinese adults. Moreover, there exist women's cadres and birth planning committees, which enable individuals to seek advice and discuss their personal problems within the setting of an informal and friendly atmosphere. China probably provides the best example of a society which radically reorganised not only its socio-economic structure but also its total ecology. This is particularly noticeable with respect to Chinese women: from being subjugated individuals who had their feet tightly bound to stifle growth, they seem to have blossomed out in all aspects of economic, political and social life (see p. 211). Their transformation throws into relief the importance of a different socio-physical environment as a pre-condition of an altogether interventive approach to life.

In the preceding argument I tried to highlight the extremely intricate interdependence between numerous demographic, economic, environmental and social variables in any one social system or sub-system. Our findings presented here clearly indicate that their traditional cultural inventory equipped the vast majority of rural poor to adapt reasonably well to their difficult and often hostile socio-physical environment. The development of new technologies facilitates a better harnessing of environmental resources to improve the satisfaction of human wants. The differential access to these new technologies accounts for much of the existing socio-economic heterogeneity in the Third World. It also helps to explain changing attitudes and different fertility behaviour among the various sub-populations.

Individuals and groups of people, who managed to benefit from productive and educational innovations, got themselves into the upward spiral of success. The opportunity to take an active part in not only shaping their own lives but also those of their descendants seems to have encouraged them to adopt an overall 'interventive approach' and to begin to plan the size of their families. By contrast, most rural dwellers remain largely unaffected by modernising influences, except for some of the new medical facilities, which helped to reduce their mortality and increased their life expectancies. Cassen, who carefully examined the evidence relating to the distribution of incomes in rural India concludes that 'for the mass of the poor, there is little sign of improvement in terms of their ability to acquire basic necessities of food, clothing, fuel, and decent housing, although some aspects of their welfare have benefited somewhat. There is some fear that, as far as concerns these necessities, the situation of the poorest has deteriorated' (1975:65). Therefore, if anything, the rural poor have had reason to become more 'accommodating' since their lives are now more than ever before at the mercy of circumstances over which they have little control. They lack the opportunity to be actively involved in shaping their destinies. Though mortality among them may have somewhat declined, the odds of generations of descendants surviving under such difficult conditions are heavily weighted against them. Therefore their continued high fertility is rational, bearing in mind that reproduction is the ultimate objective of life.

Fertility Planning

The socio-economic heterogeneity which exists - which is basically a division between the 'haves' and the 'have nots' - is often overlooked in the formulation of population programmes. This is reflected first of all in the fact that most of these programmes tend to rely on advocating the use of contraceptives and secondly in the kind of family planning services available in rural sectors. For the poorest to use contraceptives necessitates *planning* the most intimate aspect of their existence, while most other parts of their lives continue to be beyond their influence. The use of contraceptives involves planned intervention in the most fundamental human activity, i.e. the act of procreation. It seems unreasonable to expect people who have to accommodate as best they can to their socio-physical environment to plan just their sex life and the number of children they will produce. Moreover, sexual intercourse represents one of the very few activities in life which can yield pleasure and satisfaction even to the poorest, for it does not necessitate access to any environmental resource. This is another obvious fact which is frequently overlooked in the formulation of population programmes (see p. 178).

The emphasis on publicising family planning services as part of population programmes is based on the assumption that the majority of Third Worlders feel the need to reduce the size of their families and only lack the knowledge to do so. I have argued in this paper that first of all the mass of individual rural dwellers, who have so far been by-passed by modernisation, do not feel the need to reduce the number of their offpsring; secondly, those who complain about having too many children do so only *post facto* because their otherwise accommodating life puts any planned activity beyond their horizons. 'Lack of knowledge or of interest in birth control devices does not mean that couples are not interested in family limitation (70.3 per cent wanted fewer children) ... There is, however, a strong feeling that fulfilment of this desire should or must stem from divine intervention' (Driver, 1963:130). Moreover, those who manage to get onto the upward spiral of success seem automatically to become concerned about their children's future and use contraceptives of whatever type suits them best. These considerations have immediate relevance to the operation of Family Planning Programmes.

Ongoing Family Planning publicity advocates that parents and two children constitute the ideal-sized family. This appeal to the parental self-interest is based on the notion of consumer rationality which 'is deeply engrained in economic thinking. It is usually assumed that the choices that individuals are observed to make are those that leave them at least as well off as any alternative open to them' (King, 1974:78). King puts a rider to this statement by saying that even economists admit that 'impulse buying can occur, advertising can shape tastes and consumers frequently regret their choices'. The attempts to make cost/benefit calculations of children are based on this very notion of consumer rationality, which assumes that all human actions are motivated by self-interest. Our researchers found a reluctance among their informants to think of children in terms of strict costs and benefits. Similarly, *The Value of Children* study reports that 'respondents were either unable or unwilling to discuss in detailed terms the financial aspects of child rearing. Most parents appeared to have little notion of what it actually costs to raise a child, and many were reluctant to discuss children as if they were consumer goods' (Arnold, *et al.*, 1975:43). Moreover, as White points out with reference to Java, in the case of family planning, the argument that is most likely to succeed is not so much 'Limiting the number of your children will benefit *you* (an argument which may not be valid) but rather: Limiting the number of your children will benefit your children - an argument which is known to be true and therefore perhaps easily received by the generation of prospective Javanese parents who must make the crucial reproductive decisions' (forthcoming). Putting the emphasis on the adverse impact of high parental fertility on their own children's lives may help to orient people, who live by the day, to consider the future results of their present actions.

Family Planning Programmes

The main thrust of family planning programmes has been in publicising coitus-connected contraceptives (e.g. condoms) as well as devices which need pre-planning to avoid conception (e.g. I.U.D., the pill, vasectomy and sterilisation). The use of both these types of contraceptives necessitates planning, the very thing many rural people have as yet been unable to apply to other aspects of their lives.

Post-conception population control seems an area which has been largely ignored, 'despite the fact that it is probably the most widely used single method of birth control on a global basis. The most rapid birth rate declines have been associated with legislation of abortion. Japan, with the most remarkable history in this area, has done very little to study it. This could be studied by considering the fertility and birth control practice of different population strata; e.g. in Japan, before and after the legislation. The reverse spectacular doubling of Rumanian fertility in one year when legal abortion was withdrawn is a 'natural experiment' of great importance' (Freedman, 1974: 34). 'Even in 19th and 20th century Europe, a considerable part of the decline in population growth was probably mediated by abortion and child neglect' (Polgar, 1971:7). Even 'Aristotle mentioned child-exposure and abortion as suitable means of preventing an excessive number of children'. (UN, 1953:22). Devereux studied 350 pre-industrial societies and found that 'there is every indication that abortion is an absolutely universal phenomenon, and that it is impossible even to construct an imaginary social system in which no woman would ever feel at least impelled to abort' (1967:98).

The universality and frequency of abortion as a means of avoiding unwanted children is generally taken as an indication of a felt need for fertility control which the women concerned would be happier to satisfy by means of pre-planned contraception. It is in this connection that the general misunderstanding of the relevant customs and attitudes of large proportions of rural dwellers becomes most glaringly obvious. Admittedly, the frequent incidence of abortion and infanticide is a sign of a desire to avoid unwanted children, but to conclude from this that better family planning facilities will take care of the need for abortion seems all wrong. Family planning involves careful planning ahead, as the term quite rightly implies; by contrast abortion is a way of dealing *post facto* with too high fertility. 'Although most village women declare themselves to be against abortion, after having about six children the women themselves try to seek ways of terminating the pregnancy over which they may have some control, although they have no power to avoid coitus and pregnancy ... folk methods leading to abortion are entirely a woman's world' (Gould, 1969:1891).

As mentioned earlier the legalization of abortion in itself appears to bring down birth rates. This, accompanied by the availability of an effective abortive pill as soon as a woman has missed one or two menstrual periods, could be even more effective in bringing about a fertility decline. I am not aware that such a pill is already on the market, although there is the 'morning-after pill', which can work up to six days after conception and functions to prevent implantation of the ovum.

However, this too involves anticipating pregnancy on the part of the woman, rather than wait until she has her suspicions confirmed.

Singarimbun reports for Indonesia that 'there is a considerable contrast in women's attitudes to abortion in principle and their behaviour when confronted with delayed menstruation ... Herbs (*jamu*) are widely taken to induce menstruation. Herbs and tablets to bring on menstruation are widely advertised in newspapers and magazines ... Although regular menstruation is closely identified with good health, several respondents admitted that special herbs are also frequently taken by women who feared that delay in menstruation signified pregnancy'(1974: 137). In the People's Republic of China 'they use foot-pump vacuum abortion devices for any woman who wishes to terminate a pregnancy. If her previous period ended 40 days ago or more up to 70, no expensive or complicated pregnancy test is undergone. Vacuum abortion is automatic on demand' (Leonard, 1974:11). Though this means of abortion appears to be a simple and safe way to terminate an unwanted pregnancy, it does involve resorting to help from others; i.e. a midwife or a herbalist. It may prove more efficient to invest more in research concerned with producing an effective and safe abortive pill than to continue spending money on the discovery of increasingly more sophisticated contraceptive devices. As mentioned already, there is ample evidence to suggest that abortion is part of the traditional cultural inventory of most, if not all, societies. Other traditional birth control devices, as for instance post-partem taboos, may also deserve more attention. Altogether, medical research in the field of birth prevention seems to need more contact with social scientists familiar with Third World cultures. There is no *a priori* reason to believe that contraceptive devices which have been generally adopted in Western countries are automatically also acceptable to the rest of the world's populations. Socio-medical research might regard it as a challenge to produce efficient means of birth control more appropriate to Third World societies.

Conclusion

Population growth now occupies much of the thinking and discussions on development. The papers in this volume, though they represent provisional findings only, indicate that fertility behaviour is an integral part of the overall traditional cultural inventory. If this proposition is correct, and our studies seem to show that it is, it suggests important policy implications.

First of all, customary methods of birth prevention might have to be examined more carefully with a view to updating them by reducing health risks to users. This in itself may not result in greatly reduced fertility, yet it may prove more effective than many of the existing contraceptive devices. In the short run at least, population programmes might be more successful if they built more firmly on customary practices, rather than trying to innovate planned pre-coital contraception in cultures unfamiliar with such planned solutions.

Second, and more important in the long run, might be the general recognition that the overall desired decline in birth rates is unlikely to eventuate merely by improving family planning services. Yet this seems to be the main thrust of on-going anti-natal policies. A drastic change in the socio-physical environment surrounding the vast mass of Third Worlders seems essential before the majority of people begin to think in terms of fertility planning. From our studies it emerges that people need to be given the opportunity to shape their own lives, as well as those of their offspring, before they are prepared to plan the number of their children.

Finally, it should be stressed here that though such fundamental changes in the relationship between individuals and their socio-physical environment seem a necessary precondition of widespread fertility planning, they are not in themselves sufficient in ensuring declining birth rates. The Chinese experience exemplifies the need for appropriate family planning programmes supported by strong social sanctions to back up self-reliance in order to reduce population growth rates. 'Ultimately ways must be found to bring self-interest and societal interest into congruence, so that demographic events will contribute to, rather than detract from, the goal of improving the common welfare' (Arnold, *et al.* 1975:158). For this to be done effectively many more studies like our in-depth micro-level investigations and *The Value of Children* (Arnold, *et al.* 1975) surveys are required. The world is, as yet, only at the threshold of knowledge relating to fertility behaviour.

NOTES ON CONTRIBUTORS

All contributors except T. Dyson and P. Kane are currently members of the research project - A Cross-Cultural Study of Population Growth and Rural Poverty - which is being carried out at the Institute of Development Studies, Sussex, directed by Professor Epstein.

DAS GUPTA, MONICA, graduated from the London School of Economics in 1974 with B.Sc. and M.Sc. in Economics. A preliminary analysis of her fieldwork in North India was published in *Populi*, Volume 3, Number 1, under the title 'Economics, Fertility and the Green Revolution'.

DUBE, MUKUL, graduated from the Birla Institute of Technology and Science (BA) and the Delhi School of Economics (MA). He held a junior Research Fellowship at the Jawaharlal Nehru University and is currently completing his doctoral thesis at the University of Sussex. He has published jointly with T.N. Madan an analysis of twenty-five years' issues of The Eastern Anthropologist. Contributor to *The Paradox of Poverty* (see Epstein).

DYSON, TIM, graduated from the London School of Economics (B.Sc.Soc., M.Sc.Econ.) and currently a Research Fellow at the Centre for Overseas Population Studies, London School of Hygiene and Tropical Medicine. Previously Research Officer at the Institute of Development Studies, Sussex, where he carried out demographic research and acted as demographic consultant to the current research project. His recent work with R.H. Cassen on new population projections for India has been published in *Population and Development Review*, Volume 2, Number 1.

EPSTEIN, T. SCARLETT, is a Professor at the Institute of Development Studies, University of Sussex. Until 1972 she was Senior Fellow in the Department of Economics, Research School of Pacific Studies, Australian National University, where she worked since 1959, with a short break at the College of Advanced Technology, Salford, where she was Senior Lecturer in the Department of Liberal Studies. Professor Epstein has done extensive fieldwork in South India (1954-56 and 1970) and in New Guinea (1959-61 and 1967-68). She is the author of *Economic Development and Social Change in South India* (Manchester University Press, 1962), *Capitalism, Primitive and Modern - Some Aspects of Tolai Economic Growth* (Australian National University Press, 1968), *South India: Yesterday, Today and Tomorrow* (Macmillan, 1973), and has edited *Opportunity and Response - Case Studies in Economic Development* (C. Hurst & Co., 1972) as well as *The Paradox of Poverty - Socio-economic Aspects of Population Growth* (Macmillan, 1975). She has also written a number of articles and contributed to several symposia, all concerned with the problems of 'economic development and social change'. Recently she has focused her interests more narrowly on the social aspects of population growth and the role of women in rural development.

GUNASINGHE, NEWTON, received his BA and MA in Sociology from the University of Sri Lanka and Monash University respectively. Formerly Research Assistant at the University of Ceylon and Research Officer at the National Council for Higher Education in Sri Lanka, he is presently completing his D. Phil degree at the University of Sussex. Contributor to *The Paradox of Poverty*.

JACKSON, DARRELL, graduated in Sociology from the Polytechnic of Central London and is currently working as Project Co-ordinator for the Cross-Cultural Study of Population Growth and Rural Poverty at the Institute of Development Studies, Sussex University. Co-editor of the *Paradox of Poverty*.

JAIRATH, VINOD K. graduated from the Indian Institute of Technology, Kanpur, in Aeronautical Engineering in 1971 and received his MA in Sociology from the Delhi School of Economics in 1973. He is now at the University of Sussex completing his doctoral thesis. Contributor to *The Paradox of Poverty*.

KANE, PENNY, worked as a journalist for 16 years in East Africa before joining the British Family Planning Association as manager of their information and training unit. Following a period as press officer and sub-editor at the IPPF she joined the David Owen Centre for Population Studies, Cardiff, where she is currently working as technical information officer.

MKANGI, GEORGE, C.,graduated in 1971 from the University of Dar es Salaam, Tanzania, and then took up a teaching career first at Ribe Secondary School in Kenya, and subsequently as headmaster of the Aggrey High School, Kenya. He completed his MA in the Sociology of Development at the University of Sussex where he is now registered for a D. Phil degree. Contributor to *The Paradox of Poverty*.

ONWUAZOR, SAMMY N., graduated in Social Anthropology from the State University of New York in 1971, where he also worked as a research assistant. He is currently a postgraduate student at the University of Sussex, where he is completing his D. Phil degree. Contributor to *The Paradox of Poverty*.

SSENNYONGA, JOSEPH W., holds certificates in Philosophy and Theology from St. Thomas Aquinas Theological College, Uganda, and graduated in 1972 from Makerere University, Kampala (BA Sociology). He has worked with the United Nations, Kampala (FAO, PBFL) and is currently studying at the University of Sussex where he is completing his doctoral thesis. His interim field work results were published in *Populi*, Volume 3, Number 2, as 'The Cultural Determinants of Demographic Trends'. Contributor to *The Paradox of Poverty*.

TILAKARATNE, W.M., graduated from the Universities of Ceylon (B.A., Econ.,) and Kent (M.A., Econ.,) and taught at the former before joining the current research project at IDS.

BIBLIOGRAPHY

ANDORKA, RUDOLF, "The History of the Literature on the One-Child System in Southern Transdanubia", *Statisztujau Szemie*, No. 12, 1969.

ARNOLD, FRED, *et al.*, *The Value of Children*, East-West Center, Honolulu, 1975.

BAILEY, F.G., *Caste and the Economic Frontier*, Manchester University Press, Manchester, 1957.

BANKS, J.A., *Prosperity and Parenthood*, Routledge & Kegan Paul, London, 1954.

BARAN, PAUL A., *The Political Economy of Growth*, Monthly Review Press, New York, 1957.

BARCLAY, G.W., *Techniques of Population Analysis*, Wiley, New York, 1958.

BARDHAN PRANAB, K., "Some Aspects of Inequality", in Ashish Bose, *et al.*, (eds.), *Population in India's Development 1947-2000*, Vikas Publishing House, Delhi, 1974.

BECKER, GARY S., *An Economic Analysis of Fertility, Demographic and Economic Change in Developed Countries*, National Bureau of Economic Research, Princeton University Press, Princeton, 1960.

BLANCHARD, F., *Employment, Growth and Basic Needs*, International Labour Office, Geneva, 1976.

BRASS, W., *Mortality Estimation by Indirect Means*, UNESOB, Beirut, 1972.

BRASS, W., *et al.*, *The Demography of Tropical Africa*, Princeton University Press, Princeton, 1968.

CARRIER, N. AND HOBCRAFT, J., *Demographic Estimation for Developing Societies*, Population Investigation Committee, London, 1971.

CASSEN, ROBERT, *Population, Development and the Distribution of Incomes*, IDS Communication 107, Institute of Development Studies, Sussex, 1973.

CASSEN, ROBERT, "Welfare and Population: Notes on Rural India since 1960", *Population and Development Review*, Vol. 1, No. 1, 1975.

CENTRAL BUREAU OF STATISTICS, *Demographic Baseline Survey Report*, Ministry of Finance and Planning, Kenya, 1973.

CHENERY, HOLLIS, *et al.*, *Redistribution with Growth*, Oxford University Press, London, 1974.

CHERINCHOVSKY, D., *Fertility Behaviour in Developing Economies: An Investment Approach*, unpublished Ph.D. dissertation submitted to the City University of New York, 1975.

COALE, A.J., "The Demographic Transition Reconsidered", *Proceedings of the International Population Conference*, Liege, 1973.

COALE, A.J., and HOOVER, E.M., *Population Growth and Economic Development in Low Income Countries*, Princeton University Press, Princeton, 1958.

DARLING, M., *The Punjab Peasant in Prosperity and Debt*, Oxford University Press, Bombay, 1947.

DEMENY, PAUL, "Early Fertility Decline in Austria-Hungary: A Lesson in Demographic Transition", in D.V. Glass and Roger Revelle, (eds.), *Population and Social Change*, Arnold, London, 1972.

DEMENY, PAUL, "Population and Development: An Agenda for Policy-Oriented Research", in *Social Science Research and Development*, papers presented to a conference at the Ford Foundation, New York, 1974.

DEVEREUX, GEORGE, *A Study of Abortion in Primitive Societies*, Julian Press, New York, 1955.

DEVEREUX, GEORGE, "A Typological Study of Abortion in 350 Primitive, Ancient and Pre-Industrial Societies", in G. Rosen, (ed.), *Abortion in America*, Beacon Press, Boston, 1967.

DRIVER, EDWIN D., *Differential Fertility in Central India*, Princeton University Press, Princeton, 1963.

DYSON, T., *On the Relationship between Demography and Social Anthropology*, Institute of Development Studies Discussion Paper No. 68, Institute of Development Studies, Sussex, 1975.

EASTERLIN, R.A., "Toward a Socio-Economic Theory of Fertility: Survey of Recent Research on Economic Factors in American Fertility", in S.J. Behrman *et al.* (eds.), *Fertility and Family Planning: A World View*, University of Michigan, Ann Arbor, 1969.

EDWARDS, EDGAR O., "Population-Related Choices and Development Strategy", in *Social Science Research and Development*, papers presented to a conference at the Ford Foundation, New York, 1974.

ENKE, S., *Economic Development through Fewer Births*, General Electric Company, California, 1967.

EPSTEIN, T. SCARLETT and JACKSON, DARRELL, (eds.), *The Paradox of Poverty: Socio-Economic Aspects of Population Growth*, Macmillan, New Delhi, 1975.

ESPENSHADE, T.J., "The Price of Children and Socio-Economic Theories of Fertility", *Population Studies*, Vol. XXVI, No. 2., 1972.

FERNANDO, D.F.S., "Differential Fertility in Sri Lanka, *Demography*, Vol. II, No. 3, 1974.

FERNANDO, D.F.S., "Changing Nuptiality Patterns in Sri Lanka 1901-1971", *Population Studies*, Vol. 29, No. 2, 1975.

FORDE, D., and JONES, G.I., *The Ibo and Ibibio-Speaking People of South Eastern Nigeria*, International Publications Service, New York, 1962.

FRANK, GUNDER A., *Capitalism and Under-Development in Latin America*, Monthly Review Press, New York, 1969.

FREEDMAN, RONALD, "Social Research and Programs for Reducing Birth Rates", in *Social Science Research and Development*, papers presented to a conference at The Ford Foundation, New York, 1974.

GOULD, KETAYAN H., "Sex and Contraception in Sherapur - Family Planning in a North Indian Village", *Economic and Political Weekly*, Vol. IV, No. 49, 1969.

GREEN, M.M., *Igbo Village Affairs*, Frank Cass, London, 1964.

GREENWOOD, D.J., *Unrewarding Wealth,* Cambridge University Press, New York, 1976.

INTERNATIONAL LABOUR OFFICE, *Employment, Incomes and Equality*, ILO, Geneva, 1972.

JOLLY, R., "The World Employment Conference", *Futures*, Vol. 8, No. 4, 1976.

JONES, G.I., "Ibo Land Tenure, *Africa*, Vol. XIX, No. 4, 1949.

KATTI, A.P., "Characteristics of Seasonal Migrants", *Journal of the Institute for Economic Research*, Vol. 1, No. 1, 1966.

KING, TIMOTHY, "Economic Research Priorities for Population Policy", in *Social Science Research and Development*, papers presented to a conference at the Ford Foundation, New York, 1974.

KLUCKHOHN, FLORENCE ROCKWOOD and STRODTBECK, FRED. L., *Variations in Value Orientations*, Greenwood Press, Westport, Connecticut, 1973.

KUZNETS, SIMON, *Aspects of Post-World War II Growth in Less Developed Countries*, Yale University Economic Growth Center Discussion Paper No. 234, Yale, 1975.

LAWRIE, A.C., *A Gazetteer of the Central Province of Ceylon*, Government Printers, Colombo, 1896.

LEONARD, GRAHAM, *A Report for IPPF on Education for Birth Planning in China*, IPPF, London, 1974.

LEVINE, R.A., *Dreams and Deeds: Achievement Motivation in Nigeria*, University of Chicago Press, Chicago, 1966.

LEWIS, OSCAR, *Village Life in Northern India: Studies in a Delhi Village*, Vintage Books, New York, 1958.

LIPTON, M., "The International Diffusion of Technology", in *Development in a Divided World*, D. Seers and L. Joy (eds.), Penguin Books, London, 1971.

McNICHOLL, GEOFFREY, "Community-Level Population Policy: an Exploration", *Population and Development Review*, Vol. 1, No. 1, 1975.

MANDELBAUM, DAVID G., "Social Components of Indian Fertility", *Economic and Political Weekly*, Vol. VIII, Nos. 4-6, 1973.

MAULDIN, W.P., *et al.*, "A Report on Bucharest", *Studies in Family Planning*, Vol. 5, No. 4, 1974.

MEEK, C.K., *Land Law and Customs in the Colonies*, Oxford University Press, London, 1944.

MENCHER, JOAN, "Family Planning in Chingleput District, Madras, India", in Steven Polgar (ed.), *Culture and Population*, Schenkman Publishing Co. Inc., Cambridge Massachusetts, 1971.

MOLNOS, ANGELA, "The Socio-Cultural Background to Fertility and Family Planning: Analysis of 23 Studies conducted in E. Africa 1952-1970", in David Radel (ed.), *Population and Family Planning in Rural Africa*, No. 14, The African Studies Center, Michigan State University, Michigan, 1971.

MUKERJEE, R. (ed.), *Fields and Farmers in Oudh*, Longmans, London, 1929.

MYRDAL, GUNNAR, *The Challenge of World Poverty*, Allen Lane, London, 1970.

NAG, MONI, *Factors Affecting Human Fertility in Non-Industrial Societies: A Cross-Cultural Study*, Yale University Press, New Haven, 1962.

NAMBOODIRI, N.K., "Some Observations on the Economic Framework for Fertility Analysis", *Population Studies*, Vol. XXVI, No. 2, 1972.

NOTESTEIN, F.W., "The Economics of Population and Food Supplies", in *Proceedings of the Eighth International Conference of Agricultural Economists*, Oxford University Press, London, 1953.

ONWUAZOR, S.N., "Population Growth, Modernisation and Social Status among the Igbo of Nigeria", in T.S. Epstein and D. Jackson (eds.), *The Paradox of POverty*, Macmillan, New Delhi, 1975.

ONWUAZOR, S.N., "The Declining Age Grade System of Umueke: A Study in Structural and Institutional Changes", unpublished mimeo, Institute of Development Studies, Sussex, 1975.

OTTENBERG, S., "Ibo Receptivity to Change", in W.R. Bascom and M.J. Herskovits, (eds.), *Continuity and Change in African Cultures*, University of Chicago Press, Chicago, 1959.

POLGAR, STEVEN, "Culture, History and Population Dynamics", in Steven Polgar (ed.), *Culture and Population*, Schenkman Publishing Co. Inc., Cambridge, Massachussetts, 1971.

RANIS, GUSTAV, *Development Theory at Three-Quarters Century*, Yale University Economic Growth Center Discussion Paper No. 242, Yale, 1976.

ROSTOW,W.W., *The Stages of Economic Growth*, Cambridge University Press, London, 1960.

ROY, KRISHNA, "Population Policy from the Southern Perspective", in *Beyond Dependency*, G. Erb and V. Kallab (eds.), Overseas Development Council, Washington, 1975.

SEERS, DUDLEY, *The Meaning of Development*, Institute of Development Studies Communication Series No. 44, Sussex, 1969.

SIMONS, JOHN, "The Indigenous Midwife in Asia - Supporter or Opponent of Family Planning?", in *International Planned Parenthood Federation Medical Bulletin*, Vol. 9, No. 5, 1975.

SINGARIMBUN, MASRI, and MANNING, CHRIS., *Fertility and Family Planning in Mojolama*, Institute of Population Studies, Gadjah Mada University, Yogyakarta, 1974.

SRINIVAS, M.N., "The Social Structure of a Mysore Village", in M.N. Srinivas (ed.), *India's Villages*, Asia Publishing House, Bombay, 1955.

UCHENDU, V.C., *The Igbo of South East Nigeria*, Holt, Rhinehart & Winston Inc., New York, 1965.

UNITED NATIONS, *Population Bulletin No. 7*, United Nations, New York, 1965.

UNITED NATIONS, "The Determinants and Consequences of Population Trends", *Population Studies*, No. 17, 1953.

VAN VELSEN, J., "The Extended-Case Method and Situational Analysis", in A.L. Epstein, (ed.), *The Craft of Social Anthropology*, Tavistock Publications, London, 1967.

WAGNER, G., *The Bantu of North Kavirondo*, Vols. I and II, Oxford University Press, London, 1949 and 1956.

WHITCOMBE, ELIZABETH, *Agrarian Conditions in Northern India*, Vol. 1, University of California Press, Berkeley, 1972.

WHITE, BENJAMIN, "The Economic Importance of Children in a Javanese Village", in Moni Nag, (ed.), *Population and Social Organisation*, Moulton, The Hague, forthcoming.